The Love To Care

How To Take Care of Yourself with Love While Taking Care of an Aging Loved One

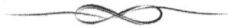

Abijah MANGA

Blandine Manga

Identifiers: ISBN: 978-1-958851-04-3 (e-book) / ISBN: 978-1-958851-03-6 (paperback) / ISBN: 978-1-958851-05-0 (Hardback) Title: The Love To Care / Description: First Edition.

Cover design by: Derek Creative

MIB Consulting LLC Control Number: 20221856975309 www.mabij.net / fondationmabij.com / lovinghomecare.net

Printed in the United States of America

MIB Consulting LLC

22 Bissette Drive, Colchester VT 05446

(802) 829-0338

info@mabij.net

To all senior citizens around the world, your life is very valuable.

And to all caregivers who have dedicated their lives to helping the elderly in need of care, your work will be unforgettable!

Special Thanks

Loving Home Care LLC sponsored this project. A Caregiving agency that provides its clients with the type of care we would want for ourselves and our loved ones.

Loving Home Care LLC aims to improve the quality of the elderly's lives by providing client-directed, compassionate, and innovative care.

Loving Home Care LLC collaborates with clients' families, physicians, discharge planners, social workers, hospice, and area visiting nurse agencies to bring a culture of caring that is cost-effective and accessible to meet each client's home care needs: Homecare, Hospice Care, and Respite Care.

For more information, visit www.lovinghomecare.net or contact them at 802-489-4927. They are at 22 Bissette Drive, Colchester, VT, 05446 - USA.

Contents

Introduction

Caring for the elderly is difficult, and older people often feel isolated in their homes. Therefore, this book aims to educate caregivers, friends, or family members on how to best care for the elderly who are struggling with any type of illness through the power of love and compassion. The book is also a must-read if you are caring for an elderly person and feel overwhelmed, lost, or simply need support in a difficult caregiving situation. Understanding the legal, psychological, technical, and spiritual aspects of caregiving is essential to helping the caregiver, and family members recognize their role and how best to help those in need.

Anyone caring for the elderly or entering the caring professionals will find this book an insight into the world of compassionate love and care. The author was a caregiver himself in his family and faced great challenges during that time. Because of his experiences, he has dedicated his life to educating others on how best to care for the elderly who need help or are on the road to recovery by writing this book.

This book provides step-by-step guidance for caring for the elderly with unstable health while maintaining their dignity and autonomy. Chapters include tips on managing burnout during caregiving, providing support and care for various common illnesses in the elderly, and, most importantly, how to best take care of yourself in the process. Because not everyone has access to quality health care or educational resources, this book is accessible to everyone, regardless of their background or socioeconomic status.

So, before you dive into this book, ask yourself if you are ready to embark on an unforgettable journey of compassion and love.

CHAPTER 1

Aging Is A Blessing

Perception of Aging around the World

Aging is a natural process that affects everyone, regardless of where they live or to what culture they belong. Some cultures see older people as wise and respected, while others associate aging with decline or loss of vitality. Often, these perceptions are based on cultural beliefs about what it means to grow old and become a senior member of society. For example, in some Asian cultures, it is ideal for older people to remain active and independent, even if their health declines. Conversely, in Western societies, aging is often associated with dependence, requiring extensive care from relatives and healthcare professionals. Regardless of how people view aging, it is clear that attitudes towards the elderly play an important role in shaping how we think about ourselves as we get older and transition into our later years.

Overall, these cultural factors can help shape individuals' growing older experiences. Though these perceptions are unlikely to change overnight, all societies need to consider how we can better support our aging citizens and ensure that all seniors feel valued and respected. By 2050, there will be almost 1.5 billion people aged 65 and over, with this percentage representing one out of every six people in the world (Report from UN DESA's Population Division).

In some places, society places a great deal of focus on youth and beauty, so older adults are seen as "past their prime" or no longer relevant. These perceptions can lead to ageism and prejudice against the elderly, leaving them feeling marginalized and isolated. Ultimately, how we perceive age is a reflection of our cultural values, making it an incredibly complex issue that varies widely from one community to the next.

Let us look at how different cultures around the world view aging in Asia, Africa, America, and Europe.

Asia

As health care and life-sustaining technology have advanced dramatically throughout Asia, the region's population has grown rapidly in a brief span of time. Almost 60% of the world's current population is made up of Asian countries, with China and India being the three most populated countries. Japan has taken the lead in Asia with the highest percentage of elderly citizens. In contrast, Bangladesh has a relatively young population, with only 3% of people aged 65 and older. This change in the population is expected to continue over the next few decades.

By 2050, Japan's elderly population is expected to reach 36%, while Bangladesh's will reach 11%. This trend is having a profound impact on both countries. For Japan, it means a shrinking workforce and increasing healthcare costs. For Bangladesh, it means more opportunities for young people as the country increasingly relies on its aging population for economic growth.

In regions of Asia where cultural norms and traditions influence the perception of aging, there is a distinct set of commonly held beliefs about old age. These beliefs typically revolve around increased passiveness, frailty, and dependence on others. For example, it is estimated in China that by 2040, 28% of the population will be over 60 years old; it is believed that the elderly are no longer able to work independently and must rely on children to support them financially.

Researchers found significant differences regarding attitudes towards older people between the East and the West. To do this, they experimented on two different samples: 184 young people from the UK and 249 young people from Taiwan. The results showed split attitudes towards older people in these cultures – some saw them as competent and admirable, while others saw them as less capable and pitiful. Interestingly, personal attitudes about older people in regard to the affective and behavioral components were more negative in Taiwan.

It has long been believed that Eastern cultures view ageing more positively than Western cultures. This is due to the influence of Confucian values, which teach respect for the elderly and promote positive views of aging. One study attempted to explore this difference by asking people from different cultures to rate how much they agreed with statements such as "older people are often wiser" and "older people should be respected." The results showed that those from Eastern cultures generally agreed more with these statements than those from Western cultures.

Additionally, many elderly people in Asia expect to retire from their roles as members of society and instead spend their days peacefully at home, free from worldly concerns or obligations. It is common for older members of Asian communities to be presenters of wisdom or knowledge and are relied upon for guidance in decision-making. As such, while aging may come with challenges unique to this part of the world, it also offers its own opportunities and rewards when viewed through an Asian lens.

Africa

Research by the University of Mkar in Nigeria found that aging is viewed as a time of wisdom and respect in African society. The elderly's opinions matter in African society, and their advice is highly valued. African cultures tend to have a more positive view of physical aging as a time of strength and experience. This positive outlook on aging contributes to the fact that many African cultures place a high value on family and community.

In traditional African societies, it was customary for families to take care of their elderly members until their dying days. This was done out of respect for the elders and their contributions to the community. There was an atmosphere of mutual sacrifice; parents made great sacrifices for their children, and their children had to make sacrifices for their elderly parents. In today's society, where older people are left to fend for themselves, this tradition has been lost for the most part.

As modernization sweeps across the African continent, traditional ways of life are changing. One of the most significant changes is how they care for the elderly. Traditionally, older people were respected and cared for by their extended family; however, with the onset of modernization, a system that supported the care of older people was lost. The modern trend has created challenges for older people.

In recent years, the majority of elderly people in African society have been isolated and put into elderly homes. Unfortunately, these homes are often underfunded and understaffed, which leads to rampant abuse of their elderly residents. They often leave the elderly without food or water and are beaten or neglected. The conditions in many of these homes are deplorable, and the elderly often suffer from malnutrition, poor hygiene, and lack of medical care.

America

In America, the perception of aging varies depending on where you live. In some parts of the country, the views of the elderly are based on experience and people's wisdom. However, in other parts of the country, ageing is viewed as a burden on society, and the elderly can be treated disrespectfully. The aging population is a problem in many countries, but Americans have been approaching this way of thinking slower.

A recent study by the Pew Research Center found that while majorities in Europe and other regions see aging populations as a pressing issue, just 46% of Americans agree with it. On the other hand, the majority of U.S. citizens believe individuals are responsible for ensuring their own financial security in old age. This is because America is one of the most affluent countries in the world, and seniors are expected to outnumber children by 2050. Despite this positive outlook on aging, there are some challenges that come with an aging population, such as medical care and support.

Europe

Aging is an unavoidable part of life, and it typically carries with it certain conceptions and stereotypes. In

Europe, these perceptions are influenced by cultural and historical factors as well as by changing social norms. Some common stereotypes of aging include the idea that older adults become less productive or capable, need more support from society, or are hard to adapt to changes. However, these assumptions may not always be accurate. For example, research shows that the average older adult in Europe remains active and engaged in social and professional life well into old age. Additionally, many European societies offer a variety of services and support to help older adults maintain their health and wellbeing.

A survey, which asked respondents to rank 25 EU countries according to their perception of discrimination against older people, found that Bulgaria and France had the highest number of people that faced age discrimination. At the other end of the scale, Denmark and Poland had the lowest level of perceived discrimination.

In Europe, the perception of ageing also varies depending on where you look. In some parts of Europe, such as Germany and Scandinavia, ageing is seen as a positive phase. They respect the elderly for their life experiences, and they are often active members of their communities. However, in other parts of Europe, such as Spain and Italy, aging is seen as the other way around, and the elderly are treated with disrespect as if they were a burden on society.

Additionally, reports suggest that young people consider older people's lives to have little value or meaning, contributing to systemic ageism in society. Despite these concerns, many experts argue that encouraging positive attitudes towards aging will lead to better outcomes for older adults and younger generations. Through initiatives such as intergenerational mentoring programs and empowering lifelong learning opportunities, it starts to change perceptions about aging and its impact on the world. In short, happiness and satisfaction in life come from within, no matter what your status in society may be.

How to Consider the Elderly

When it comes to caring for the elderly, there are many considerations to consider. As people age, they experience changes in their physical and cognitive abilities. Depending on a person's functional capacity, they may need assistance with basic tasks like cooking and cleaning or more complex tasks like managing finances or paying bills. Many older adults may struggle with mobility issues and require assistive devices like canes or walkers.

When interacting with elderly individuals, it is important to be patient and understanding, as they may have difficulty communicating or remembering things. Finally, it is critical to consider the needs of the elderly when providing care and to recognize that they are intellectual and valuable members of society. Treating each situation with care and respect makes a positive difference in their golden years.

We will explore these topics more as we consider how to embrace the elderly among us in any society.

Accept them for who they are

It can be difficult for older people to feel accepted in a world where the youth are more valued. Embrace the elderly with respect to their opinions and ideas. You need to stop thinking of them as living in the past or out of touch with modern culture. They might not understand everything going on now, but that does not mean they are not interested in learning about it. They have lived through tough times we can only imagine, and their stories are filled with rich details from which you could learn a lot.

Everyone wants a companion

Many elderly people can live independently with greater ease than ever before. However, if your senior citizen lives independently, they are likely to feel lonely and depressed. Make an effort to check in on them once or twice a week, ask about how they are doing, and catch up for coffee—and make sure you give them plenty of advance notice before you stop by.

Be respectful but not patronizing

When dealing with an older person, it is important to be respectful but not condescending. You do not have to use baby talk or treat them as if they are incapable of doing simple tasks. Your tone should be warm and inviting to make them feel respected as individuals in society with an equal amount of power in their conversation.

Go slow and get permission

Remember that going slow is essential, whether it is someone you already know or someone you just met. Do not overwhelm them with attention; ask permission before making any physical contact to avoid any offense. If they seem welcoming to your affection, ask how they want to be approached and let them guide you accordingly. Understand their unique needs, whether that means listening to what they say or letting them talk through tough things without judgement.

Life Lessons through an elderly lens

Many people see the elderly as nothing more than a drain on resources. However, this thinking is shortsighted and fails to consider the valuable role that the elderly can play in society. The elderly have a wealth of experience and knowledge that will benefit society as a whole. With their years came decades of experience and life lessons. They want nothing more than to share them with younger generations. Rather than rejecting and shutting them out or ignoring them, recognize what they have to offer and learn from their experiences.

Discover How to Live Your Best Life as You Age

You know that your body and mind change as you age, but did you know that your attitude, interests, and activities can change too? These changes can be good or bad, depending on how you react and view them. If you accept these changes with open arms, you can learn to make the most of your aging life. The tips below will help you do just that so that even at the end of your days when you retire from your career and spend more time at home, you will not have to settle for just surviving.

The Importance of Knowing Yourself

One of the biggest challenges for older adults is not discovering who they really are. Now is a great time to start if you have not discovered yourself yet. Some helpful ways to learn about yourself are by discovering new hobbies, joining a local group, getting involved with charity work, or journaling. Ask family members questions about what you were like when you were younger and see if there are any similarities between then and now. This technique will help you know yourself from a broader perspective; you can then highlight your characteristics in bullet points and focus on the things that make you happy.

The 3 Pillars of Successful Aging

Research has found that to live out your life with optimal wellness, there are three pillars of successful aging: physical fitness, mental health, and positive social relationships. Adhering to these principles sets you up for longer and healthier life. Here is what they mean and how to put them into practice.

1. Physical Fitness

Our hearts can only take so much, and exercise strengthens cardiac function. However, not any type of exercise will do – aerobic activity is key. Aerobic exercises increase heart rate over an extended period, improving blood flow through small blood vessels in our extremities and organs; walking 30 minutes per week meets government recommendations for seniors. One study found that seniors who walked 20 minutes 3 days per week enjoyed significant boosts in both cognitive and motor functions over 2 years; they were also half as likely to suffer from a fall injury during that time period as those who didn't walk regularly.

Being physically active is important for maintaining health and longevity; it also increases endorphin levels, reducing stress and making you happier. The saying "use it or lose it" applies here – by staying active now, you will prevent having to increase your physical activity level as you age. It helps maintain muscle mass, prevents bone loss, improves balance and coordination (reducing the risk of falls), and boosts mood and energy levels. Exercising can take many forms, such as walking, biking, or yoga—find something that suits your lifestyle and schedule best. Not only will you be able to stay active while enjoying yourself, but it also helps to ward off depression, which increases with age due to changes in brain chemistry related to age-related illnesses like Alzheimer's disease.

2. Staying active mentally

The brain tends to shrink as you age, but there are ways to counteract some of those effects. Learning new skills or just reading something new can help challenge your brain, which in turn keeps it functioning better for longer periods. Think back to what made you happy when you were younger, whether it was playing sports or taking piano lessons. It may be hard to remember exactly why these activities gave you joy. Still, if you think about all of your interests over time, eventually, something will stand out as something that would still give you pleasure today if given another chance. If nothing else comes to mind, look into classes at local colleges or continuing education programs through adult education centers—chances are good that someone somewhere is offering an activity similar to one that brought you happiness before.

3. Fostering relationships:

Social relationships become more valuable in old age, so try to create positive memories with friends and family. Having people around you whom you love and care about gives your life meaning even when times get tough. Maintaining contact with loved ones does not mean seeing them every day – making phone calls or sending emails/text messages is often easier for older adults and cheaper than visiting faraway places (especially after paying for travel expenses). Keeping track of birthdays and other important dates lets the people you care about know how much you appreciate them.

Creating a Joyful Aging Path

As you age, the world can seem to get smaller. You may leave your career and friends behind and find it harder to stay active and involved in your community. It is normal to feel like you are losing control over your life as you age. However, there are ways to create a joyful ageing path for yourself that will help you keep feeling engaged and connected throughout your later years.

1. **Spend less money (or save it):** Money doesn't buy happiness. Still, it allows you freedom from worry, so choosing a frugal living path isn't

necessarily bad, depending on what matters most to you personally. By spending less, you can put more away for your future and avoid accumulating debt that could cause problems down the road. While it is true that life is short and to spend not to worry about finances, it is also true that you need to make a comfortable living and, therefore, need to earn enough to cover basic needs. Spending wisely can help you achieve both goals—but only if you are honest with yourself about your priorities.

2. **Make sure your home is safe**: Whether or not you plan to sell it, it is still a wise idea to make sure it is safe for potential buyers who might want to see it during open houses or when they come by for showings. Falling is one of the most common accidents for seniors and is a hazard in homes that are not equipped with proper safety features. Making sure your home is safe from falls can help you age in peace and maintain independence as long as possible.

3. **Take care of your body:** Your body will change as you age, but there are still things you can do to make it last longer, be healthier and function better throughout life. A healthy diet made up of fruits, vegetables, whole grains, and lean protein

helps reduce the risk of diseases such as stroke, heart disease, and diabetes.

4. **Don't compare yourself to others:** A lot of things in life are relative, and aging is no exception. There is no judgment regarding how we age — each person ages differently based on genetics, lifestyle choices, and a host of other factors. Just because your neighbor is more successful than you or your high school friend appears younger does not mean they are better off than you. Be proud of what you can do and enjoy yourself to the fullest.

5. **Take care of your skin:** As you age, your skin becomes thinner and less elastic. It is also more susceptible to damage from UV rays. Use sunscreen daily and avoid sunlight exposure during peak hours (between 11 a.m. and noon). Consider using anti-aging products that improve the appearance of wrinkles and fine lines.

As you age, finding things that make you happy is important. For some people, that might mean spending more time with their family; for others, it might mean traveling or taking up a new hobby. Whatever brings you joy, make time for it in your life.

Find Happiness in Your Golden Years How to Exercise, Meditate, and Eat For Success

While most of us would do anything to stop time and stay young forever, we have to come to terms with the fact that, barring any super-advanced medical breakthroughs, we are still going to age and get older. This does not have to be the end of the world; instead of thinking about how old you are getting, you can focus on improving your health and happiness in your golden years by exercising regularly, meditating frequently, and eating healthily.

Exercise

Yes, it is that time again—getting up early so you can fit a workout into your day. Research has shown that exercise helps prevent chronic diseases such as heart disease and diabetes and contributes to well-being by improving sleep quality. Finding an activity, you enjoy, whether dancing, hiking, swimming, or playing tennis, is key. Regular physical activity lowers blood pressure and cholesterol levels, increases HDL (good) cholesterol levels, and helps prevent osteoporosis in women after menopause.

In addition to aerobic exercise, try strength training at least twice a week to build muscle mass and increase bone density. Strength training also makes everyday tasks easier by building stronger muscles in your arms, legs, back, and core. For those over 50 years old or with medical conditions, it is best to talk to your doctor before starting any new exercise routine.

Meditation

Meditation is a practice that yields myriad health benefits. A 2017 study found that people who practiced Transcendental Meditation daily experienced significantly lower stress levels. Another study published in 2018 found that mindfulness meditation reduced inflammation in people with rheumatoid arthritis. Meditation proves to help ease anxiety and depression symptoms. As a bonus, regular meditation may even slow down age-related cognitive decline. Studies show that meditating just 30 minutes a day could slow the brain's aging by up to 10 years.

There are several different ways you can approach meditation. Some techniques focus on calming and quieting your mind; others involve visualizations or mantras, and others require you to keep focused while sitting still or performing specific exercises. Whether you treat it as a matter of stress reduction and clearing your mind or as a way of strengthening concentration and focusing on yourself, meditation is something that can benefit almost anyone. Meditation becomes a powerful way to achieve silence and harmony in one's life, find one that works best for you and give it a shot.

Diet

When you take care of your body, it will take care of you back. Eating a healthy diet can boost happiness and help prevent health issues later. To maintain a healthy weight as you age, consider cutting down on red meat (which contains saturated fat) while increasing the consumption of fish (which is high in protein). Incorporating plenty of fruits, vegetables, and whole grains into your diet can help boost energy levels, improve moods, and keep your body functioning at its best. Try not to skip meals; eating regularly helps control hunger cravings, so you do not overeat later. It also keeps your metabolism going strong.

Aging can often feel like a death sentence, but while you are still alive, there is no reason not to be happy. Finding happiness is not about chasing fleeting experiences or trying to be perpetually optimistic—it comes from finding joy in everything you do. If you prioritize happiness, you will find it even as you age. Aging is truly an opportunity to discover happiness with a new exercise, meditation, and diet regimens. You can enjoy many more golden years with just a few small changes in your lifestyle. What are you waiting for? Start today!

Don't Stop Dreaming How to Keep Hope Alive as You Age

As people age, they often find that their hopes and dreams change. For some, this means reconsidering what they want to do with their lives. For others, it may mean coming to terms with the fact that certain goals are no longer possible. However, aging can also be an opportunity to develop new hopes and dreams. This may involve taking up a new hobby or reconnecting with old friends. It can also be an opportunity to set new goals and get closer to achieving them. Whatever the case, aging provides a unique chance for people to reflect on what they want out of life and make positive changes. Here are some ways to keep hope alive as you age.

Surround yourself with positive people: To keep your hopes and dreams alive, you must believe that things will improve. To do so effectively, you need to maintain connections with people. Having people around you who care about your well-being will always help you stay positive and hopeful. Engaging in new activities or trying something you have never done before is great for keeping those hopes alive because it keeps the mind working, which helps prevent stagnation.

Appreciate your worth: A lot of pressure is placed on adults to succeed and make a fortune. But your worth shouldn't be defined by what you have or what you make—it should be measured by how well you treat others, how you keep yourself challenged, and whether or not you're living up to your full potential. Do not let social pressure discourage you from going after your dreams; embrace them and know that they do not define who you are.

Be involved in getting old: As you get older, your attitude towards society and culture changes. If you isolate yourself socially and culturally, it can lead to despair and sadness. A study from AARP revealed that those who had no interest in activities outside of their home often felt they aged much faster than those who participated in their communities. Those surrounded by happy memories felt younger than those who focused on negativity. So be sure to keep up with friends, family, and hobbies — it will keep you adventurous.

Hope gives you something to strive for and keeps you motivated to achieve your goal. It is also a source of comfort during difficult times. When you are facing challenges, remembering your hopes and dreams can give you the strength to move forward. Hope is a powerful belief that will lead you to new dreams, inspire you to achieve great things, and help you survive the storms of life.

The Hidden Gifts of Aging Opportunity To Give, Share, And Be Close To Nature

While many people view the process of aging with dread and fear, you need to shift your perspective to see it as an opportunity to give, share, and be closer to nature. As you grow older, you gain a wealth of knowledge and experience that is priceless. You become more aware of what matters most to you, both mentally and emotionally. This allows you to connect with others on a deeper level and offer your wisdom to those in need. Some possibilities include volunteering at your local shelter or serving as a docent at the local historical society. For example, if you're an experienced cook or baker who loves teaching others how to prepare delicious meals at home, consider joining a local cooking class where you can share your knowledge with others while gaining new friendships. People can benefit from your extra time and energy, but only if you do not let it go to waste.

In a recent study by the University of Texas at Austin, researchers found that people over 64 years old who were able to share their knowledge and wisdom with younger generations felt more confident and satisfied with their lives. This study also showed that when older adults share what they have learned from life, they can feel more connected with others and less isolated.

As you age, your brain is still capable of learning and growing. You can use that knowledge to help others. For example, many retired professionals continue working part-time jobs because they enjoy socializing with co-workers or helping others in need while also making some extra money.

On the other hand, ageing gradually makes you more attuned to your natural surroundings and can connect you with the rhythms of nature in a meaningful way. You begin to reflect on your life with rose-colored glasses, remembering the best parts with clarity and forgetting the not-so-good parts altogether. This can be especially true when looking at nature. It seems to bring about feelings of nostalgia in its many forms, whether it is beautiful cherry blossoms on an early spring day or snowfall that blankets trees and sidewalks alike in the middle of winter as you spend time with nature, from gardening and hiking to simply sitting in a park or forest and listening to the sounds of the wind in the trees. Whatever your chosen method may be, allowing yourself to connect with nature at this stage in life can enrich your sense of joy and improve your overall health and well-being.

If you are ready for a new adventure that embraces all life offers, do not fear aging—embrace it. By sharing your gifts with those around you and reconnecting with the beauty of nature on a deeper level, you can find true meaning and happiness even at difficult times.

How to Provide Care and Comfort to an Aging Person

As people get older, their bodies change, requiring more assistance than when they were younger. Often, this means that they need help from family and friends to perform daily activities such as eating or getting dressed. While this assistance is important for maintaining their physical health, it is also important to provide mental care that helps to eliminate loneliness and sadness and promotes emotional support. Here are some ways you can provide care to an aging person:

- Encourage social interaction by planning outings or visits with family and friends.

- Make sure the individual has access to transportation.

- Spend time talking with the individual about their life experiences. This can help them to feel connected to others and provide an opportunity to share wisdom and knowledge.

- Help the person stay active by participating in activities together or helping them to access resources such as senior centers or fitness classes.

- Encourage emotional support by doing things together, like playing board games, going for walks, reading, or watching movies.

- Ensure that your parent or grandparent has access to medical care and support from professionals.

- Encourage the expression of feelings by listening openly and nonjudgmentally. This can help the individual feel valued and understood.

By providing care with a focus on social, emotional, and physical needs, you can help an aging person live a happy, healthy, and fulfilling life. By providing emotional support and focusing on their well-being, you can help them age with happiness and contentment. By putting your loved one's needs first, you can ensure that they remain healthy and happy for years to come.

It takes a special kind of person to become a caregiver who makes a difference in people's lives. In the next chapter, you will learn how ordinary people answer the call of being a caregiver, balancing their personal lives and careers as caregivers, and the challenges and rewards that come along with it.

Key takeaway

1. Some cultures see older people as wise and respected, while others associate aging with declining or losing vitality. The perception of aging is based on a country's cultural, historical, and social beliefs.

2. To embrace the elderly include being full of patience, care, and acceptance of who they are.

3. To live your aging life means discovering your inner self deeply.

4. The three pillars of successful aging ensure you live a thriving and meaningful life.

5. Creating a joyful aging path includes minimizing materialism and enjoying the moment with loved ones.

6. The key to aging gracefully is taking good care of yourself and enjoying a healthy, active lifestyle.

7. Instead of worrying about how old you are, focus on how you can improve your health and happiness.

8. Practicing meditation daily unlocks your life's harmony.

9. Hope keeps the soul young and inspires you to achieve great things.

10. The hidden gifts of aging include a deeper understanding of life, a greater sense of purpose and self-awareness, and the ability to share knowledge and experience with others.

11. You can find peace and solace by spending more time in nature and contributing back to society.

CHAPTER 2

Why We Become Caregivers

❧

Compassion, Empathy, and the Drive to Help Others

The International Alliance of Carer Organizations (IACO) report estimated that there are more than 63 million caregivers internationally. In the United States alone, more than one in five adults are caregivers, and the number is increasing as the elderly population continues to rise.

Caregiving can be a challenging but rewarding experience. There are many reasons why people become caregivers, but the most common factor is the nature of human beings. As social creatures, we are driven by our desire to help others and become part of something bigger than ourselves. For some people, this desire is so strong that they choose to become caregiving professionals, dedicating their careers to helping others in ways that go beyond what friends and family can provide.

What does it mean to be a caregiver? What are the attitudes and behaviors that define this role?

One key component of being a caregiver is the willingness to provide care, which includes having an attitude of readiness to help whenever needed. This willingness can manifest in many ways. For example, caregivers may quickly offer assistance when they see someone struggling, even if they are not directly involved in the situation—by checking in on them regularly or making themselves available for support if needed.

Researchers Zarzycki and Morrison surveyed various caregivers' driving motivations for caregiving. They found that many people choose to become caregivers out of love and a sense of obligation rather than out of a desire for financial gain or professional recognition. Many caregivers are driven by the desire to provide high-quality care and maintain companionship with their loved ones. In fact, many caregivers find great satisfaction in their roles and believe that no one else is available to provide the same level of care as they do.

In general, there are two primary types of motivation for providing care: extrinsic and intrinsic. Extrinsic motivation is driven by external factors such as the desire for social recognition or the desire to meet perceived social expectations. While intrinsic motivation comes from within oneself and is driven by a sense of fulfillment and satisfaction that is felt while engaged in caregiving, in either case, intrinsic motivation is the main reason why people choose to become caregivers.

One factor in how people perceive aging is their culture's attitude towards informal caregiving. The term "informal caregiving" refers to unpaid care to a family member or acquaintance with a long-term health or care need. In cultures where informal caregiving is valued, aging is viewed as a time of growth and contribution. In contrast, in cultures where informal caregiving is not valued, aging is viewed as a time of decline and dependency. Another feature of how people perceive aging is their personal experience with aging. Those who have had positive experiences with aging are more likely to see it in a positive light, while those who have had negative experiences are more likely to see it negatively.

In short, caregivers motivated by love and affection provide better support to those in their care. Whether it is helping with personal hygiene, providing meals, or simply being there for company, these unsung heroes make a real difference in the lives of others.

Sudden Caregivers Learning to Care for Loved Ones

A sudden caregiver is anyone whose life is drastically changed by the need to care for a loved one with an unexpected diagnosis. Caregiving can be overwhelming, and it often surprises people who never considered themselves caregivers. In a 2015 study, about one in ten adults aged 40 and older with a parent aged 65 or older provides sudden care for a parent. It is comprised of 5% of younger adults and 14% of older adults.

Suppose you have recently become responsible for the care of an older parent, spouse, or another family member. In that case, you may feel overwhelmed at the thought of suddenly taking on this responsibility. You might also worry about how you will handle the situation financially, emotionally, and logistically — especially if a loved one has special needs or you live far away from home. If so, you are not alone; about 43 million caregivers provide unpaid care, and this book will help you overcome and handle the challenges you face along the way.

At the beginning of the journey, it can be overwhelming. There is no way to predict how many people are calling you, expecting that you will take care of them. All of these added responsibilities can make it difficult to complete everyday tasks and remain productive at work. It is important that you do not neglect your own needs in order to take care of others. Being informed and prepared for what is to come can make you mentally ready for the new responsibility of being a sudden caregiver. Here is what you will be encountering as a sudden caregiver:

The Physical Impacts of Having an Ill Family Member

You may have to care for a family member who is suddenly incapacitated. If your loved one has a terminal disease or is in physical pain due to an injury, they will require your attention and help with everyday activities like bathing, eating, and walking. You may have to administer medications and monitor vital signs. The healing process can be long and exhausting if a family member has suffered an injury that leaves them with significant physical limitations, such as amputation or paraplegia.

The Mental Challenges of Taking Care of an Ill Family Member

It is a challenge on its own to take care of yourself, but when you suddenly find yourself caring for an ill loved one, it adds new emotional stressors to your life. Before taking on responsibilities such as bathing, cooking, and helping with transportation, it is important to consider how these new roles may affect your emotional well-being. These challenges can have an adverse effect on your mental health if you are not prepared beforehand. You might not be able to get in a good workout at home because much more work needs to be done—and that work is physically demanding. If you struggle to balance your personal fitness goals with those of your family members, you might need to rethink how to create more time for yourself.

Dealing with Your Own Feelings

When you are dealing with new, stressful responsibilities, it can be hard to figure out what you are feeling. One of your first steps should be sitting down and making a list of how you feel and why. Once you have that information written down, consider which situations make those feelings worse or better and why they affect you so strongly.

Situations like these are important to know because they could help shape how your family takes care of themselves. For example, if taking care of yourself is difficult when you are at work but easier when you are alone at home, then having a caregiver come in after work might be an option worth considering. You do not need to have all your answers right away; it might take months or years before everything falls into place. Nevertheless, understanding where you stand now will give insight into how to move forward in a way that makes sense for everyone involved.

The Challenges of Being A Caregiver

Caregiving is a difficult, stressful, and often thankless role. As the care recipient's needs become more complex and demanding, you may struggle to meet them. Especially when the task you are performing is the one you like to do, and the person you are caring for does not appreciate your efforts. In a 2018 survey, 33.1% of older adults' unpaid caregivers reported experiencing some sort of adverse mental or behavioral health problem; moreover, 27.6% of them reported having a major depressive disorder.

There are many trials associated with being a caregiver. Still, by learning about these challenges ahead of time, you can get the support you need from family members, friends, and other community resources to succeed as a caregiver. You may also find yourself feeling overwhelmed by the responsibility. Here are some tips for dealing with your emotions as a caregiver:

Keeping your own life in order

The hardest part of being a caregiver is keeping your own life in order. It is important to remember that you are not just a caregiver—you are also a human being with needs. You have to make sure you can care for the other person by taking care of yourself first. Keeping organized is one way to balance your responsibilities as a caregiver; for example, if you have children, it might be helpful to set up a calendar where you can track when you will take them on outings or spend time with them after school. This way, you do not have to rush through any important tasks at work or neglect any other obligations in your personal life.

Making time for yourself could mean taking a walk around the block during lunchtime or meeting up with friends for lunch every couple of weeks so you can catch up without worrying about cooking dinner or cleaning up afterward. It could also mean setting aside time to read or watch your favorite TV show each day. With just 15 minutes, a relaxing break can help clear your mind so that you can handle things better when things start getting hectic down the road.

Managing emotional stress

Try to control your anger towards the elderly or yourself for not being able to do everything in your way. Caregivers can feel frustrated when they think about how much time they spend on caregiving tasks and what they miss out on in life. As a result, you may feel guilty if you do not have time for your friends or activities that used to bring joy into your life. Not beating yourself up over these feelings is important because it will only worsen things. Here are some tips to help you cope with frustration.

- **Be aware of your own emotions.** You have every right to feel stress, anger, and frustration when caring for someone sick or elderly. However, if you do not know what is happening inside yourself, it will be harder for you to work through those feelings healthily.

- **Set boundaries with family members**. It is natural for other people in the house to help with the caregiving duties, but if they are doing too much or not doing enough, it can add to your stress levels. Be sure everyone knows their responsibilities, so everyone feels like they are contributing equally.

- **Do not take things personally**. It may seem like it's all about you because it's happening to your loved one—but remember that caregivers often get stressed because they feel like they're not being heard or respected by others around them (even if they're not saying anything). Ignore what people say about you and always focus on being on the positive side—you will save yourself a lot of trouble down the road!

Physical burnout from overwork or injury

Physical burnout from overwork or injury is a common problem among caregivers. Burnout is characterized by physical and emotional exhaustion, including symptoms like insomnia, depression, irritability, lack of appetite, restlessness, and anxiety. If you are feeling these symptoms, it is time to take a step back from your responsibilities as a caregiver and take some time for yourself.

Caregivers often have trouble prioritizing their own needs and getting time for themselves outside of caring for others. This can lead to burnout and exhaustion, leading to more stress and anxiety about properly caring for your loved one. Here are some ways to make sure that you are doing the best job possible for your loved one while also taking care of yourself:

- Take breaks, especially if you are feeling overwhelmed or burned out. You can even schedule time off without worrying about missing work or being away from your loved one.

- Make time for self-care activities in between breaks, such as exercise and meditation, to charge your energy.

- Explain to the people around you what it is like to be a caregiver so they support you when needed and do not pressure you into doing more than what feels right for your situation.

- Do not try to do everything yourself because this will only make things worse for you and the patient. Instead, focus on what you can do best by dividing tasks among those who live nearby so that everyone gets some rest when needed without having too much work piled up at once.

- If possible, try using technology such as video conferencing apps instead of visiting in person; this will save time and energy for everyone involved in planning visits with loved ones who are far away from home (or even just across town).

- Avoid Isolation. Being isolated from other people can lead to feelings of depression, which makes it harder for you to do your job well. Try volunteering at a local organization or joining a community group to meet new people who share your interests.

Feeling overwhelmed, underappreciated, alone and isolated

Feeling overwhelmed, underappreciated, alone, and isolated are the various phases of being a caregiver. It is vital to recognize these challenges and learn how to cope with them so that you can stay strong. However, being a caregiver is more than just a job; it is a commitment to love and care for another person.

It can be especially hard if you have other children or family members who need your full attention. You may be doing everything you can to take care of everyone else while still managing to stay healthy yourself—but the stress of the situation can take a toll on both your mind and body. Here are some suggestions on how to cope with these challenges:

- Take care of yourself first before taking care of others. Caregivers often neglect themselves because they are focused on caring for someone else. Make sure that you take time out for yourself and engage in activities that make you happy, such as reading, exercising, or doing puzzles. These activities will help relieve stress while also keeping your mind sharp, which will be beneficial when caring for others who may need assistance with certain tasks.

- Start a gratitude journal for all of the things that make your life worth living.

- Book regular time off for yourself, so it does not feel like a luxury when you do take time off— make it part of your routine.

- Remember that everyone needs support sometimes—no matter what his or her circumstances are. Take advantage of local resources like senior centers or community organizations offering support groups and classes on managing stress during hard times.

Don'ts

- Do not hide your feelings from the people around you. It may feel too much to talk about how much you're struggling with something as simple as taking care of yourself—let alone someone else— but getting it out in the open will help everyone understand what's happening. You do not have to go into detail if that makes it too hard; just let them know that you are struggling and ask for their support.

- Do not compare yourself with other caregivers or think about how much better they seem to handle things than you do. Everyone struggles with different life situations despite showing only the best side.

Financial strain from work absences or paying for care

You may find yourself missing work and having to pay for essentials that can be expensive and difficult to manage, also known as financial strain. Many caregivers have to take time off work to care for their loved ones, which can result in lost wages or using up all of their vacation and sick days. Additionally, if you are paying for care, it can be expensive, depending on how much help you need.

Caregivers may also struggle with medical bills if their loved ones are living in long-term care facilities or have home health aides who come into their homes regularly. Governmental programs like Medicare only cover certain levels of care; many caregivers find themselves paying out-of-pocket for these services and other medical services not covered by insurance.

You must adjust your lifestyle and budget if you care for someone who depends on you. Caregivers often have to make difficult choices about whether to work or to care for their loved ones. Taking time off work to care for a family member can mean lost wages, while paying for outside care becomes increasingly costly as the need increases.

As a caregiver, you need to find support that helps you cope with these challenges. Financial assistance may be available through local government programs or private organizations. It is important to find out what financial resources are available before deciding how to pay for care.

These adjustments might include:

- Exclude paying for extra services like housekeeping or laundry.

- Be transparent with your employer; let them know your circumstances. It is important they know so they can help adjust your schedule and payments accordingly.

- If you cannot get support from your employer, look into applying for disability or unemployment benefits.

- Consider taking advantage of short-term disability benefits. This will allow you to take time off without risking losing income or insurance coverage.

- Apply for assistance programs like the Supplemental Nutrition Assistance Program (SNAP) or Medicaid Benefits Program, which provide food stamps and health insurance coverage. These programs are available to low-income individuals with disabilities or illnesses.

They will help cover some of the costs associated with providing care for a loved one.

- Ask for help from your social circle, friends, or family members for basic tasks like cooking meals or cleaning.

How to Be a Good Caregiver

There are so many ways to be a good caregiver, and it is not always easy to figure out the best route. Luckily, you can benefit from the experiences of others who have already figured this out. This guide will help you understand what a good caregiver looks like in different situations. Caregiving skills do not come naturally to many people. Still, it is something that you often need to learn to make the elderly thrive and feel comfortable in their situation with your assistance. Here are some qualities you need to develop:

Put yourself in their shoes.

To be a good caregiver, you need to put yourself in the shoes of your elderly patient and try to understand their situation. You need to be compassionate and understanding when they are having a bad day and ensure they get all the help they need.

When you are taking care of an elderly person, it is easy to get frustrated with their inability to do things for themselves. You may feel like they are being stubborn or difficult. However, remember that they were once able to do everything by themselves, and now they cannot. They might not even know how much they need help—they just want to be independent, so they try to do everything on their own and end up hurting themselves.

You should also take note of any changes in behavior that may appear over time, such as depression, dementia, or confusion due to dementia (which is common among older adults). These conditions can cause trouble for caregivers because these symptoms can lead to violent behavior towards others, including loved ones or caregivers themselves. Caregivers need to recognize these symptoms early on so they can address them before things get worse. When you are dealing with an elderly person who is resistant to your attempts at helping them out, it is a good idea to take a step back and breathe deeply before talking again. Give them time to think about what you have said before continuing the conversation, so they can adjust their perspective on things if necessary.

By putting yourself in their shoes. Imagine what it would be like if your body was failing and needed constant care. *What would make your life easier? What would make it harder?*

Be compassionate and understanding of their needs and limitations. You cannot expect your loved one's condition to improve overnight—it takes time for them to heal and get better. However, you can help them feel comfortable, safe, and in control of their lives so they can feel their best as quickly as possible.

Be a good listener

Being a good listener to an elderly person is one of the best things you can do to help them feel valued, important, and cared for. Elderly people feel like they do not matter as much as they did when they were younger. The key here is to actively listen to them. Active listening is a way of paying attention to what another person is saying and responding with comments that show you are paying attention. It alleviates these feelings and demonstrates to the elderly that they are of value. For example, if someone says, *"I love chocolate ice cream,"* you might respond by saying, *"That's great! You must enjoy it a lot."*

Here are some other tips for active listening:

- Be patient. It may take an elderly adult longer than usual to say what she wants to say because of memory problems or difficulty communicating.

- By making eye contact and nodding your head occasionally, you show attention and interest in what the person is saying.

- Do not interrupt the person (unless it's an emergency) until she finishes speaking; if you interrupt her, she may be unable to remember what she will say next.

Be patient and mindful of elderly triggers

As a caregiver, you are often the first to know when your loved one is feeling triggered. It is important to be patient and mindful of these triggers so that you can help them get back on track and reduce the chances of a major episode.

What exactly is a trigger? A trigger is any external or internal stimulus that prompts an old memory or feeling to resurface. This can cause your loved one to become anxious or upset quickly, which may lead to an episode. If your loved one is having trouble calming down after an episode like this, it may help if you remind yourself that there is nothing wrong with taking a break from the situation if it becomes too much for either of you.

Common triggers include:

- Being in a crowded space (e.g., in a grocery store)
- Being touched unexpectedly (e.g., by someone who doesn't know them)
- Being asked difficult questions (e.g., about their condition)
- Being confused about where they are (e.g., if they've been moved somewhere new without warning)

When you are with an elderly person, remember that you are dealing with someone who has been through a lot in life. As such, being patient and mindful of their triggers is important. If they mention something upsetting, try not to get defensive or lash out at them in anger—this could make them feel like their feelings are not valid or worth listening to (and this is especially true if they are in a nursing home). Instead, just acknowledge what they are saying and let them know that you hear them; next, do your best to move on from there without dwelling on it too much.

For example, some seniors are very sensitive to noise. If you are talking loudly or having a conversation next to them, it can be extremely disruptive to their ability to enjoy their meal or use the restroom in peace. Be aware of your volume level when speaking with someone who may be hard of hearing.

In addition, many seniors have trouble seeing well when asked questions like "*how much for this?*" or "*what do I owe?*" They need more time and assistance than most people realize. Give them time to think about your question before answering—and do not rush them if they need more time than usual. They may not be able to communicate as clearly as they used to, or they may have lost interest in talking about anything other than the weather and their favorite TV shows. They may also have trouble hearing what you are saying, so speak slowly and clearly. If there are any changes in their behavior, take note of them, but do not jump to conclusions without considering all possible causes first.

Being informed About the Patient's Particular Disease

Caregiving is a lot of work, and it can be exhausting. Sometimes it feels like you are just a step behind the patient—and that step is always getting bigger. Whether the patient has Alzheimer's or cancer, your job as a caregiver is to ensure they are comfortable and their needs are being met.

The first thing you need to do is to learn how to care for the patient's particular disease. If they have Alzheimer's, read up on what symptoms to look out for (Chapter 4), what changes might happen in the future, and how to help them cope with it. If they have cancer, find out what treatments they are getting and what side effects they might experience from those treatments. Then try to plan ahead so that you can help them avoid those side effects.

It is important to stay educated and up-to-date on the patient's particular disease. A good caregiver will be able to help their loved ones in many ways, including managing their symptoms, preventing complications, and helping them get back to their normal routine. You may feel like there's nothing you can do to help someone with cancer or diabetes, but caring for these conditions isn't just about keeping them comfortable; it's also about making sure they have everything they need to stay safe and healthy while living with their condition.

Be a companion to your loved one, not just a caregiver

As a caregiver, getting caught up in the day-to-day tasks of caring for your loved one or elderly parent can be easy. You might be helping them bathe, eat, and go to the bathroom—but are you mentally there for them?

Take time to sit down and talk with them about their life. Learn about their favorite foods, books, and music. Ask about their childhood and what they wish they could have done differently. Listen as they tell stories of when they were young and healthy—and then take them out for ice cream!

Being a companion means more than just giving someone food and water; it means being present in their world in a way that makes them feel cared for and supported. Get past the fact that your loved one is older than you are and has different interests than you do. If you approach this from a place of understanding, then it will be easier for both of you to get along and enjoy each other's company.

Don't Make Promises You Can't Keep

If you make a promise to yourself that you do not keep, you lose your credibility with yourself and with others too. Promises are hard; they require effort, discipline, and a lot of time and energy. The elderly are notoriously fussy about their living conditions. If you mention bringing fresh flowers to their room every week, ensure you fulfill your words. If one of them starts complaining about how much they miss their garden at home, do not just tell them, "*oh well,*" but make the time to take them out into the garden yourself.

So how do we avoid making these kinds of promises in the first place? Let us look at some strategies:

- Think carefully before making any promises — particularly ones that involve other people.

- Try using phrases like "*I'm going to try my best*" or "*I'm working on it*" instead of saying "*Yes*" when someone asks if you will do something for them. That way, there is no pressure on either side if anything comes up and prevents one from following through on their end of things.

Set Boundaries

Boundaries help everyone feel safe and comfortable. When you work with elderly clients, set boundaries for yourself and them; if you are taking care of a loved one, guide them when they can do things and when they need to rest. Set up systems like alarms, which will remind them when it is time for their medication or just ask them if they want anything when they wake up in the morning.

It is important to you to set boundaries for yourself, you may be tempted to always be there for your loved one, but this could lead to burnout or even depression on your end. The best you can do is take breaks and spend time doing things that make you happy. For example, if you want to go out with your friends one night but your grandpa wants to spend time with you, tell him that it is important for you to spend time with your friends, too. It is fine if he responds with anger or sadness—he may not understand why it is important right away. You can explain it by stating politely, *"I love spending time with you, but I need some time alone sometimes."* You can also tell him how much fun it is when he visits his friends or goes on trips without his family. That might make him feel better about letting go of some control over your relationship.

No matter what happens in any situation, there is always a way out. You do not need to fight or argue if someone gets upset; just walk away from the situation and take some deep breaths until everyone calms down again. Setting boundaries with the elderly is a tricky thing. You want to be respectful and polite, but you also want to ensure that you are taking care of yourself, even if you have a possessive family.

Here are some things you can do:

- Set limits on how often they can call or text you to avoid distractions during work.

- Ask them not to interrupt work time or family time when they reach out to talk with you.

- Set a time limit on how long you will spend in the house each day. If it is too overwhelming, try doing one task at a time instead of trying to get everything done at once.

- Make sure you get enough sleep. It is easy to lose track when you do not get "me-time," but it is crucial for your health and well-being as well as theirs.

- Avoid asking yourself questions like "*Why am I doing this?*" or "*Why does this person insist on eating nothing but butter?*" — it will only make you feel worse about things than if you did not know anything about their habits.

- Set boundaries for yourself as a caregiver; you may want to limit the number of hours per day you spend taking care of someone else's needs so you can have time for yourself.

Grieving a Loved One How to Cope With the Emotional Loss

Losing a loved one, especially someone you have known most of your life, can be a difficult experience to endure. These emotions can be overwhelming, whether it be lost from an accident, a child, or a pet. Many have difficulty managing these emotions, especially if they are sudden or unexpected. Even though you may feel like you are alone, know that you are not alone on this journey. Others are feeling the same way as you, and there is always support available to help you manage those emotions.

Being forced to face the grim reality that your loved one will not return is tough to comprehend, let alone accept. Grieving is a natural process that helps you come to terms with their death. Processing grief is difficult if you do not know how to handle it. The physical and emotional symptoms are not easy to manage and take a lot of time to pass. Unfortunately, for some people, the grieving process can appear never-ending.

After someone you care about passes away, you go through an emotional process called mourning, which allows you to grieve and come to terms with your loss. Mourning is an emotionally and physically demanding experience; it is normal for you not only to feel sad but also angry, frightened, confused, and frustrated. You may have trouble functioning daily as you grapple with grief. If you are going through a difficult time of mourning, here are some ways you can cope if a loved one passes away and move forward.

Surround Yourself with Family and Friends

You need people around you who love and support you. If there is no one in your circle with whom you can share your grief, reach out to someone else who has been through what you are currently experiencing. This can help validate your feelings and make you feel more connected. Grief is a process that takes time, be patient with yourself as you go through it. There is no right way to grieve. Do not expect yourself to snap out of it or try not to cry because you think you should feel better by now. There will be days when you want nothing more than to wallow in your sadness—this is a natural response. Do not beat yourself up; it takes time and mental support from people around you to heal completely.

Visualize Your Loved One

Some people believe that when they lose someone they love, they will be able to see them again someday—in heaven, in a dream, or in another form. That's why many mourners like to keep photographs of their lost ones nearby. If you cannot bring yourself to look at pictures of your loved one for whatever reason, try drawing or painting him or her; some people find that using different mediums helps them feel closer. Take comfort in imagining what your loved one would say if he or she were still alive today. Would he/she give you advice? Would he/she tell you not to worry about something? You may never know exactly what he/she would say, but it is comforting to think about what kind of support and encouragement he/she might offer.

Reach Out for Help

You will likely find yourself suddenly saddled with grief when your loved one dies. You may not be able to handle some of your regular daily tasks. If you do not feel comfortable coping with all of your feelings alone, you must reach out for help. Many communities offer support groups for those who are grieving with online therapists who specialize in helping people deal with death and loss. Do not hesitate to ask friends or family members for assistance if you need it. It can also help to talk to the clergy or other religious leaders for spiritual advice and comfort.

Have an Open Heart

Grief can leave you feeling alone and hopeless, but having an open heart is one of the most important steps in overcoming it. Take time to consider what your loved one would want for you and how they would want you to move forward and be happy. Grief can change how we think about our own lives—it teaches us that there are some things we cannot control and live life more meaningfully. As difficult as it may seem, try to focus on these positive aspects of grief rather than letting yourself get lost in anger or sadness. Having an open heart will help you find strength when you need it most.

Do Not Isolate Yourself

What is important during times of deep emotional loss? Companionship. People are more inclined to grieve when alone—their loved ones and friends can help them through difficult times. If you find yourself grieving, do not isolate yourself. Reach out to your closest loved ones, as they will be able to provide support and companionship as you cope with your loss.

Green Therapy

Nature can be a healing teacher. The beach, the mountains, parks, and even being in your backyard are all-powerful places to find solace and peace when life brings heartache. Also known as "Green Therapy," spending time in nature can help overcome grief. Studies show that walking in nature can lower stress levels by reducing cortisol levels, heart rate, and blood pressure. Spending time in green environments improves moods and wellbeing. Attending a meditation class or volunteering at an animal rescue are two other ways of connecting with nature that can help you heal from a loss.

Let Go of Blame and Anger

Anger and blame can be very tempting when you are grieving, but it is important to remind yourself that these negative emotions do not serve you in any way. By holding onto them, you are not only allowing yourself time for healing but also risk alienating friends and family who are trying their best to support you. Instead of assigning blame, be open about your feelings and focus on controlling your negative emotions. This can help you start moving forward and express what you are going through to others.

Try Guided Imagery or Meditation Techniques

Even if you are not spiritual, Guided Imagery or meditation can help you find peace in your time of mourning. Guided imagery and meditation are best practiced in sessions with an expert, but they can also be used alone to help you relax. Connecting with your loved ones through these techniques might make it easier for you to come to terms with their passing. This technique helps keep your mind off their death and focuses on remembering their life and what made them special. It will help you remember all of those good times instead of dwelling on how much you miss them. If you want to learn more about meditation, check out "The Beginner's Guide to Meditation" by Dr. Andrew Weil and "The Art of Happiness at Work" by Dalai Lama.

The Rewards of Caregiving Why Giving of Yourself is the Best Way to Live

In a world where people spend more time caring for themselves, a compassionate caregiver's dedication to their family, friends, and community is priceless. Caring for people who are unable to care for themselves is one of the biggest joys you can have in life. When you love being a caregiver and let yourself get into the mindset of caregiving – truly loving it as a way of life – you will likely experience an entirely new side of your own personality you never knew existed.

In a study involving 60 family caregivers of mentally ill patients in Germany, 57% of caregivers found that the benefits they experienced were an increase in gratitude and affection from their patients, increased self-esteem and hope, self-respect, and greater inner strength. In addition, younger caregivers gained greater confidence and experienced more character development than older caregivers. Caregiving requires a special kind of person — a giver, someone full of love and compassion who takes pleasure in seeing others happy.

As you get older, you will find that caregivers increases in demand. With an aging population, it is hard to ignore the number of seniors needing help with daily living activities. When you are caring for someone who needs your help, it can be difficult to find the motivation to continue, especially when you are in an unfamiliar situation with new challenges on a daily basis. Nevertheless, taking care of others does not have to be overwhelming—it can actually be rewarding.

Here are just some of the rewards of being a caregiver so that you know what to expect when entering this role in your life:

Caregiving Gives You Opportunities To Make A Difference.

Caregiving for a loved one can be a rewarding experience and an opportunity to give back. As a caregiver, you have a chance to help others who are going through similar experiences with their own loved ones. You meet new people who share similar interests and concerns about their family members or friends. You see your actions influencing their lives. You feel like it's all worth it—the sleepless nights, the stressful days, and all the other challenges of being a caregiver—when you see how much joy your caregiving brings to another person.

It is not always easy to see the fruits of your labor and know that you have made a difference in someone's life. When people come into your life as caregivers, they often become family members. Therefore, it can be hard for both sides to leave this world because you have grown so close over time. However, it is fulfilling to know that even if someone leaves this world prematurely, they had someone who cared about them while they were living their last years. When you are a caregiver, you greatly impact someone's life. You may feel like you are giving up a lot of your own time and freedom, but the fact is that your presence makes all the difference in their lives.

Caregiving Can Give You Purpose and Direction

Many caregivers report that they feel more valued when they help their loved ones. While caring for someone else may put some pressure on your shoulders, it also gives you direction in life and helps you feel like you are making a difference in other people's lives. That kind of feeling can be very rewarding and satisfying—and it may even improve your mental health. The act of caregiving results in lower stress levels and increases overall wellbeing and happiness, making you feel needed and appreciated.

Caregivers often describe the experience as humbling, rewarding, and even empowering. Many people feel a sense of accomplishment by taking on this role. They feel like helping their loved ones live their final days with dignity and comfort.

When you are caring for someone who needs assistance with daily activities like bathing or walking around their home, you are helping them maintain their independence and dignity. When you are caring for someone who needs help managing their finances or medical information, you are helping them preserve their quality of life. Lastly, when caring for someone at risk of falling prey to elder abuse or neglect, you're preserving their safety and well-being—and that is the most wholesome action in the world.

Caregiving is the perfect opportunity to develop new skills and strengths.

Being a caregiver will help you discover your strengths and weaknesses and who you are deep inside. You will learn how much patience you have, how far your kindness goes, and what type of personality you have, and this self-discovery process will help you become a better version of yourself.

By taking on caregiver responsibilities for a loved one, you can be eligible for public benefits like Medicaid and Social Security or even qualify for part-time jobs with flexible hours. Regardless of your reasons, being a caregiver offers many benefits in both tangible and intangible ways—from better sleep at night to increased social interaction with other caregivers and care recipients alike. Despite the hardships, it is an opportunity to grow as a person and develop new skills, strengths, and abilities. Sometimes, caregiving duties can be laborious, and many forget to focus on what they are gaining from it. However, many good things come with being a caregiver, such as:

- You have the chance to spend time with someone you love while they are still around.

- You have the chance to learn about a new field— whether it is medicine or another area of healthcare—and become more knowledgeable about it.

- You get to do something important for someone else, which makes him or her feel valued and loved.

- You can use this time as an opportunity to reflect on your own life and make changes based on what you have learned from caring for someone else.

Caregiving exposes you to new people and experiences.

It is easy to be stuck in the same routine, but one of the biggest benefits of caregiving is that it forces you out of your comfort zone and into new situations. As you meet new people and learn how to help them with their specific needs, you will develop more meaningful relationships than any other kind you have had before.

Being a caregiver is not all about the patient. You will be exposed to new people, experiences, and emotions that can broaden your horizons and deepen your relationships with those you help. Caregiving can also help you better understand what it is like to go through a tough time and see things from another person's perspective. As a caregiver, you will get to know many new people and develop long-lasting relationships. You will also be part of some unexpected situations, which can help you learn more about life and love than you ever thought possible.

Though caregiving can be stressful, it can also be deeply rewarding if you approach it with an open mind and heart. Caregiving enables you to build deeper relationships with the people you love while also better understanding what they are going through.

Caregiving Boosts Empathy and Compassion

Becoming a caregiver opens your eyes, heart, and mind to a completely new world. Not only will you understand how it feels to need care, but you will also be able to empathize with those in need. Performing basic tasks for your loved one will teach you compassion and to put yourself aside for others. You will experience joy in seeing someone's face light up after you help or support them in making their bed or cooking their favorite meal.

Caring for someone else also helps you appreciate your own life and the people in it. It can help you see that many things are out of your control—and yet, even if you do not have control over certain things, there are still things that you can do to make your life and the patient's life better.

When you care for others, you are forced to acknowledge their needs and desires and see life from their perspective, making you a compassionate person. It teaches you to listen more closely than ever before—to put aside your problems and focus on someone else's struggles. To be there for them in whatever capacity they require, physically or emotionally.

While the experience may be challenging—you might feel exhausted, frustrated, or even angry—it also requires you to dig deep inside yourself and find reserves of strength within you.

How to Get Started as a Certified Caregiver

Caregivers are an essential part of the healthcare industry. They provide a crucial service to patients, families, and staff members alike. Their responsibilities include providing emotional support, physical care, and assistance with daily tasks such as bathing and eating. The caregiver also helps run errands and perform light household chores. You might work with people who have disabilities or chronic illnesses, or you might be helping seniors live independently. Caregivers may work in a variety of settings, including hospitals, nursing homes, and adult daycare centers. They may also work in private homes as domestic employees or caregivers.

A person can become a caregiver with little to no experience in this field by completing training programs that focus on the specific skills needed for the type of role. This training occurs at community colleges, health organizations, or vocational schools that offer courses on becoming a caregiver.

The general qualities required to become a caregiver include having good interpersonal skills as well as being able to provide emotional support for others. You need to manage stress to avoid being overwhelmed when dealing with difficult situations such as death.

In order to become a caregiver (which differs from state to state), one must first complete high school and obtain an associate's degree or certificate from an accredited college or university program that trains people in this field. After college or a technical school, you can get a license from your state's Department of Health Services that lets you legally work as a caregiver in that state.

The Types of Caregivers and Responsibilities

The caregiving role varies across countries or states. There are six domains involved in caregiving: daily living tasks, physical health and personal self-care, social connections, advocacy and communication with health and human services workers, monitoring and safety issues, and providing emotional support. Each domain has multiple subdomains involving professional roles, such as a caregiver's awareness of physical changes or the need to inform a loved one's doctor. Some of the most common ones include:

- **Home health assistants.** They provide personal care and other health-related services such as administering medication and assisting with daily living activities.

- **Personal care assistants.** They help people with bathing, dressing, eating, and other personal hygiene tasks. They may also assist with transportation to appointments and running errands. These workers usually work in their clients' homes and can be hired by family members or by agencies on behalf of families who need assistance caring for their loved ones but cannot afford to hire someone full-time.

- **Nursing assistants.** They help patients bathe, dress, feed themselves, and perform other tasks that require physical assistance from another person. They also provide companionship to patients at the hospital or at home recovering from surgery or illness.

Once you have decided to take the wonderful journey of becoming a caregiver, the next stage is to understand the terms commonly used in care facilities. Whatever level of care you choose to provide, learning the fundamental terms discussed in the next chapter can help you provide better care and support to your patients.

KEY TAKEAWAY:

1. When you care for someone, you see their struggles, triumphs, and heartbreaks, making you more empathetic and compassionate toward other people.

2. Giving yourself to care for others will expand your life in ways you might never have imagined.

3. Caregiving is a unique field full of opportunities to impact someone else's life while getting a chance to know people from their perspective.

4. Caregiving is a chance for you to feel like you matter most in your loved one's life.

5. Caregiving is not for the faint of heart. It can be draining, stressful, and heartbreaking, but also incredibly rewarding—both for you and for the person you are caring for.

6. Caring for someone else can give you a new appreciation for your own life.

7. Caregiving teaches you patience, compassion, and empathy at a deeper level.

8. Caregiving is a chance to grow because you have to learn new skills and adapt to new situations.

CHAPTER 3

Understanding The Basics Of Long-Term Care Facilities

～～～

Long-term care facilities provide a safe and healthy place where a patient with any kind of illness can receive the attention they need. Many types of long-term care facilities include nursing homes, assisted living homes, memory care, hospice care, and home care. These facilities offer different levels of care depending on the needs of the patient. There are over 4.7 million people employed in the health care industry in the United States.

Long-term care facilities aim to help people live as independently as possible while still receiving appropriate medical attention when needed. They provide help for those who need personal assistance with routine needs and medical supervision due to old age, disability, or an illness with no cure. Long-term care facilities (LTCFs) offer high-quality living and opportunities for personal growth, making them the first choice for many seniors.

Long-term care facilities offer a combination of healthcare services, social activities, and assistance with everyday tasks. Many people are hesitant to put their loved ones in long-term care facilities because they think it means giving up on them, but this is false. Long-term care facilities can provide excellent care for patients with various illnesses and have staff members who will help monitor your loved one's health and assist with any emergency. They provide a place where people can live out their final days with dignity, comfort, and respect.

There are many factors to consider when thinking about sending your loved one to a long-term facility. The first is whether they are ready to accept long-term facilities. If they are still able to live on their own, then they are best served by staying in their own home.

Working in Long-term care facilities

As a caregiver, you will need to learn how to communicate with residents and other caregivers at the long-term care facility. There are different types of medicine that are prescribed for patients in these facilities. You must have an understanding of the illness to best assist patients under your supervision. For example, there are different ways to help children or adults with developmental disabilities or mental illness.

If you do not have experience working in a long-term care facility, then here are some tips for caregivers to get started:

- Be prepared for shifts lasting up to 12 hours at a time. This can mean working at night or during the day, depending on the facility's schedule.

- Work under pressure and deal with challenging situations such as trying to calm down an angry resident or keeping track of medications when there are multiple residents who all need medication at once.

- Long-term caregiving facilities are located in different types of buildings and areas, but they all offer a very similar set of services:

- Dining options

- A place to sleep

- Transportation services (to get you to appointments or other activities)

- Activities like exercise classes or games

- Staff members who help with tasks like bathing, dressing, and grooming.

Not all long-term care facilities are the same. The services offered, the length of stay and even the cost vary widely depending on the facility. Long-term care facilities are broadly divided into five categories, nursing homes, assisted living, memory care, hospice care, and home-based.

Nursing Home

A nursing home is a facility that is equipped with trained personnel that takes care of a patient or the elderly under constant supervision. These are generally larger facilities providing intensive medical care, licensed nurses, and doctors. They also provide rehabilitation services for people recovering from an illness or injury. The majority of patients with Alzheimer's or dementia live in nursing homes. According to researchers' estimation, 75% of Alzheimer's disease patients who survive to age 70 will reside in a nursing home by age 80. There are over 15 thousand nursing homes in the United States, and the majority are certified by Medicare and Medicaid.

How to recognize the good one?

Generally, there are many nursing homes, but not all of them can be trusted. To find out which nursing home you can trust, you should do some research on them first. You can check their website or ask your friends who have experience with this kind of facility. A good nursing home will have a caring staff, good food, and many activities for the residents to participate in. Some things to look for in a reputable nursing home include:

- Highly trained staff.
- Cleanliness
- A variety of activities and events
- A good reputation in the community

Cost of Nursing Homes

The cost of sending your loved one to a nursing home varies depending on the services they will provide for you and how long you will be staying there. A one-month stay in a good nursing home can cost anywhere from $5000 to $9,000, depending on the location and size of the room provided to each patient. This cost increases by about 3% annually. Nursing homes can be expensive, but most insurance policies will cover at least part of the cost. It is important to note that this will likely not cover all expenses. It is best to discuss with the family members how much money they have saved up for such an event and what kind of care would work best for them financially.

The Pros and Cons of Nursing Homes

You should note that not all nursing homes are equal when providing quality service for their patients. Some may have poor sanitation systems or lack qualified medical staff, which could lead to infection and the death of their patients.

Pros:

- Staff is trained to provide medical care, including in emergencies.
- The staff is friendly, and the atmosphere is pleasant.

- The rooms are large, with lots of space for furniture.

- There are many activities available for residents and their families. These can include walking groups, art classes, and more.

- Most nursing homes have gardens, and some even have farms where residents can spend time growing vegetables or livestock.

Cons:

- The food quality can be average.

- The cost is expensive, and finding insurance that covers nursing home care may be difficult.

- Limited visitation hours with family members can be stressful for the patient and their families.

- Not all nursing homes are safe; some have had problems with neglect and abuse of residents by staff members or other residents.

Assisted Living

Assisted living is a type of housing for seniors that provides them with a variety of services and amenities. These services include meals, housekeeping, transportation to medical appointments, and more. Assisted living is not the same as nursing home care. Nursing homes offer medical care and supervision around the clock, while assisted living facilities are only open during certain hours.

Assisted living is a great option for seniors who do not need intensive care but do need some assistance with their daily activities. Assisted living communities provide a safe and stable environment in which seniors can live independently while having access to the help they need. They are licensed by the state, which means they must meet certain standards set by their respective state.

Cost of Assisted living health care

In 2020, the average monthly cost for assisted living residences was around $4,429 per month or $53,148 annually. The cost of assisted living increased by an average of 3.6% annually between 2015 and 2020.

How to recognize the good one?

The best way to find out if an assisted living facility is good is to talk with people who live there. Find out what they like about their home and what issues they are facing. Ask them if they have any complaints about the staff or other residents. You can call different facilities and ask some questions about what kind of services are offered, how many meals per day are provided (usually three), and how much it costs per month, so you get an idea about what kind of place might work best for your loved one's needs.

Look at the number of residents in the facility—if there are more than 50 residents, this may not be the best option for your loved one because more people mean more noise and distractions. Consider other factors like whether the building has an elevator or wheelchair accessibility, how close it is to their favorite restaurants or shops, if there are activities planned throughout the week (such as exercise classes), and if there is transportation available for doctor's appointments or errands like grocery shopping.

The Pros and Cons of Assisted Living Homes

Pros:

- Elderly people can meet new friends and get involved in social activities.

- Assisted living facilities provide meals and housekeeping services, which means that residents do not have to worry about these tasks when they move into an assisted living facility.

- The cost of living in an assisted living facility is less than other forms of senior housing such as nursing homes or memory care facilities, making it easier for families to afford their loved ones' care needs.

- They can enjoy fun activities like playing cards with friends over lunchtime every day rather than spending all day alone at home.

- You can get a private room, a separate kitchen, or a bathroom. Most facilities offer private rooms for residents who prefer not to have roommates.

Cons:

- Fewer services are available at assisted living facilities than at nursing homes or centers.

- Residents may feel isolated if they do not have visitors or participate in the community activities offered by the facility.

- Assisted living does not provide medical care round the clock.

Memory Care

Memory care is a type of senior care specifically designed to help people with memory loss and other cognitive issues. This can be due to dementia, Alzheimer's disease, or other condition affecting memory. The goal is to help them live as independently as possible while also maintaining their quality of life and happiness. A doctor or other health professional includes assessments of the person's memory, referrals to resources for help with their diseases, and memory training. It also includes anything from coaching people through their daily routines to helping them stay engaged with activities they enjoy.

In memory care, the staff helps residents stay on schedule with meals, activities, and other events to keep their daily routine varied. Memory care facilities have all kinds of safety measures in place to prevent dementia patients from wandering, which include alarmed doors, elevators with codes, and enclosed outdoor spaces.

How to recognize the good one?

The best way to find a good memory care provider is by asking friends, family members, or your doctor for recommendations. You should also look for state agencies that license these facilities and check out the facility's website for more information. A good place to start is by checking out online reviews, especially on sites such as Yelp and Google Reviews. You can also visit the facility in person if possible, get a tour of the building, and speak with staff members about their policies and procedures for handling emergencies and other situations that may arise during visits by family members or friends.

During your search, consider these points:

- Is the facility clean?
- Are the doors and directions clearly labeled to help residents find their way?

- Ask how they manage patients with severe dementia or aggression.

- How does the staff motivate patients to eat food?

How much does it cost?

Memory care costs depend on several factors, including where you live and which services you need. In general, however, these facilities tend to be more expensive than other types of senior housing because they offer around-the-clock support and care. Memory care facilities may also offer additional amenities such as transportation to doctors' appointments or social activities at nearby parks or shopping centers. The average memory care rent can cost around $6,000 to $7,000 per month.

Pros:

- Receive 24/7 care from trained professionals.

- Access to regular physical therapy sessions and other activities that help with cognitive function.

- Able to visit your parents anytime during normal business hours and on holidays and weekends.

Cons:

- The costs associated with memory care are much higher than assisted living or other senior housing options.

- Some patients may find that they do not like the way their new environment is and are reluctant to stay.

Hospice care

Hospice care is a special kind of end-of-life care for terminally ill people. It focuses on improving the quality of life for patients by providing comfort and relief from pain, stress, and emotional distress. Hospice care is available to people with any type, stage of illness, or disease. The goal of hospice care is to give comfort and help while taking into account what the patient and their family want.

Hospice care is designed to support families through difficult times. For example, hospice professionals may help you plan for end-of-life arrangements such as funeral services and burial locations. They can also help you talk about your feelings surrounding death with your family members and friends and provide support for those who are grieving the loss of a loved one. It can help people who are dying and their families who may be experiencing pain or other symptoms associated with the dying process.

Hospice programs generally provide 24/7 access to nurses and other health professionals who can help with pain management techniques like meditation or breathing exercises; this allows patients' quality of life to remain high despite their physical condition deteriorating over time due to their illness progression.

Hospice care is not only for those with 6 months or less left to live; it can be used earlier in the disease progression when the patient's condition has worsened significantly, but he or she is still able to communicate his or her wishes regarding treatment options. The doctor will help you determine whether hospice care is appropriate for your loved one based on his or her needs and preferences.

How to recognize the good one?

When choosing hospice care, there are many things you can look out for that will help you identify whether they provide high-quality care. Here are some things to consider:

1) Does the hospice have a license? A license means they can legally provide hospice services in your state. If this is important to you, ask about their licensing status before agreeing on any terms or signing paperwork with them.

2) What does their website say about them? Good places will often have information about their staff structure, mission statement, and even patient testimonials available online so potential clients can get an idea about their services.

3) The best way to recognize good hospice care is to look for a provider that has an in-depth knowledge of your loved one's condition and history and can offer you personalized care plans based on their specific needs and concerns. You should also look for providers that provide access to multiple treatment options, including medications and physical therapy.

Cost of Hospice care

It is important to recognize high-quality hospice health care because it is possible to receive high-quality palliative care without paying expensive premiums. For instance, some hospices may charge more than others because they provide additional services like transportation or housing assistance. However, some hospices may also offer these services at no additional cost.

Hospice costs vary depending on where you live and how much care you need, but most plans will include medications and medical supplies for up to six months. The Medicare service can pay for most of the service, costing around $10,000 per month.

Pros:

- Monitor and provide 24/7 care to patients.
- Reduces stress on the patient and family.

- Provides comfort to patients who are suffering from pain or discomfort.

- Providers can often remain with patients longer than in traditional nursing homes, which helps them develop trust in their care providers.

- Helping patients and their families cope with the emotional aspects of death.

- Providing physical, emotional, psychological, spiritual, and social support through education, counseling services, and support groups.

- Patients can stay in the same place they feel comfortable with instead of moving to a new environment.

Cons:

- Costs are often higher than other types of end-of-life care like hospitalization or home care services.

- Not always covered by insurance companies.

- Sometimes families do not want their loved ones to go into hospice care because they feel like they are giving up on them.

- Hospice care focuses on palliative (end-of-life) care rather than curative (life-prolonging) treatment options—which means that patients who have been given only months or weeks left to live may not receive treatments that could extend their lives significantly longer.

At Home Care

At Home Care provides care and assistive services to older adults and people with disabilities at their homes. Depending on the patient's needs, they can provide care 24/7 or some hours.

Home care is an option for seniors and their families who may need some assistance with daily tasks but do not want to move into a long-term health facility. At Home Care aims to create a safe environment by providing the patient with the support they need to live independently at home. They assist with daily living activities such as bathing, dressing, meal preparation, and personal care like shaving or hair styling. Home Care agencies also offer companionship services such as reading books aloud or writing letters for those who are unable to do so on their own.

How to find a good home care agency?

You can search for home care agencies on the internet, in phone directories, or ask your friends or relatives who may know some good agencies. You can also contact your local Area Agency on Aging. They will help you find an agency in your area that offers different kinds of services at different costs. When looking at different home care agencies, there are several things you should ask about before deciding on one.

- Ask the agency what type of training they offer their employees and how often they provide updates on new techniques or procedures.

- Ask if they have any programs that support clients with chronic conditions like diabetes or heart disease—these are often overlooked by other agencies but can make all the difference when it comes to helping seniors stay healthy.

- Get references from friends or family members who have used that particular agency before, so you can find out if it was a positive experience for them as well.

How to recognize the good one?

If you are considering hiring a home care professional, make sure they are licensed by the state and bonded. You should also ask if they have any complaints against them filed with the state licensing agency or complaints filed with the Better Business Bureau (BBB). The BBB should be able to tell you if there have been any complaints against them within the last 2 years.

Costs of Home Care

The cost of at-home care varies from state to state and from agency to agency because each has its own policies regarding how much time clients spend with caregivers each week, month, or year.

Pros:

- Patients get to stay in their familiar surroundings and get the care they need close to home.

- You do not have to worry about whether or not your loved one is getting the right care. The caregiver will be qualified, licensed, bonded, and insured.

- It is easier to schedule appointments at home than in a hospital or nursing home.

- Cheaper since you get to pay per hour for the service.

Cons:

- Privacy concerns, it can be hard for family members to watch someone else move around their house and keep track of their belongings.

- There is less oversight during at-home care, so there are higher risks of abuse and neglect.

Planning for Long-Term Care

In the United States, the average person will spend an estimated $12,000 on long-term care, with almost 7.5 million Americans having long-term care insurance.

Long-term care is a broad term that covers a wide range of services, including health care, home care, and residential care. Long-term care can affect anyone at any age and stage of life. People need long-term care mainly due to an illness or disability that limits their ability to perform daily tasks. Mental illness and dementia can also lead to the need for long-term care, along with physical disabilities.

It is important to think about how your situation will change as you get older and whether your current living situation will support your old age. For example, suppose you have a family history of Alzheimer's disease or other forms of dementia. In that case, it might be worth considering an assisted living community where you can receive assistance with tasks such as bathing and dressing. If you do not have much money saved up and are worried about how much longer you will be able to afford your current home, it may be worth looking into a senior apartment building that offers subsidized rent for seniors. If you want to stay in control of your finances but need more help around the house than friends or family members can consider hiring an in-home caregiver who can cook, clean, shop for groceries, or assist with personal care needs.

Whatever option seems best for you, planning now will help ensure that when the time comes, you do not have to rely fully on family or friends for your health expenses. Planning for long-term care means considering options available to you so you can take steps to protect your assets and preserve your independence. There are alternatives to long-term care insurance for covering the expense of long-term care if you do not have it. You can look into Medicaid and Medicare, which are government programs that provide help with paying for long-term care expenses. The requirements vary from state to state, so it is important to look into your status and state eligibility.

Differences between Medicaid, Medicare, and Long-term Insurances.

Medicaid, Medicare, and long-term insurance are all government-run health insurance plans that help people pay for their health care necessities. Each has different criteria, but they all have the same goal: to get you the care you need without paying full price.

The biggest difference between Medicaid and Medicare is who can qualify for them. Both are intended to cover low-income individuals, people with disabilities, and families who may not be able to afford other health care coverage options.

Medicaid

The states administer Medicaid. Medicaid is for low-income people who do not have much money saved up for their health care needs. In order to qualify for

Medicaid, most states require you to be disabled or have children under 18 living in your home who are disabled or have special needs. Medicaid covers many services, such as outpatient care, prescription drugs, hospice care, long-term care services, transportation to medical appointments, eye exams and glasses, dental treatment, and mental health services. Statistics show that Medicaid represents 43% of long-term care spending while Medicare is at around 21%.

Medicare

Medicare works a little differently than Medicaid because anyone over 65 can qualify regardless of their income or assets. Medicare also counts the disabled and individuals that reach end-stage renal disease. Medicare is a social insurance program managed by the federal government that helps to pay for the cost of hospital care, physician services, lab tests, and prescription drugs. The benefits are paid by Social Security taxes, which are deducted from each paycheck or paycheck stub. Medicare has a lot more coverage options than Medicaid but does not cover long-term care in nursing homes.

Both programs are available to those over 65 years old or disabled people who meet certain income requirements. Both programs offer comprehensive health coverage. That means they provide all types of medical services, from hospital care to prescription drugs to mental health care. You can still apply for both if you have a disability or a serious illness, even if you are on Social Security Disability Insurance (SSDI).

Long-Term Health Insurance

Long-term care insurance protects you or your loved one from the high cost of long-term care services and supports you by paying for at least some part of your expenses in a nursing home or assisted living facility, depending on the services you choose. Normally, long-term health insurance is divided into groups and individuals.

Group long-term health insurance is issued through an employer or other group plan administrator on behalf of employees or members. Individual long-term health insurance is purchased directly from an insurance company. It is usually purchased by self-employed or unemployed people who do not have access to group coverage through an employer. Individual long-term health insurance is often more expensive than group coverage because it does not have the same economies of scale as group plans. The main advantage of individual long-term health insurance is that it provides better coverage than short-term health plans, which may only last for three months or less.

Long-term health insurance policies are common in the United States, but there are some important things to consider when considering long-term health insurance.

- If your employer offers group coverage, you might want to take advantage of it instead of trying to get insurance on your own.

- When choosing a long-term health insurance policy, make sure the policy covers what is important to you in terms of services and costs. Some policies may have limits for specific types of treatment or equipment; make sure that any policy you choose provides comprehensive coverage that meets your needs.

- Understand what types of expenses are covered by your long-term health insurance. Many policies come with exclusions like Medicare payments (if eligible), prescription drugs (if eligible), dental care (if eligible), vision care (if eligible), and other medical expenses not directly related to long-term care, such as routine physicals and check-ups;

Key Takeaways:

- When deciding about long-term care, it is important to consider what your goals are and how you want to live out the rest of your life. If you are still working and want to stay active and engaged in the world, you might want to consider a long-term care plan that allows you to live independently at home.

- If you are ready for a more relaxed lifestyle but still want to remain connected with friends and family, assisted living or home care could be the right choice for you.

- If you need more intensive care and help with daily tasks like bathing or eating, you can get care around the clock at a nursing home or memory care facility.

- Each health care facility has its pros and cons— and they all require specific considerations before making final decisions about how best to proceed.

- Medicare is managed by the federal government and provides health care to citizens over 65 years of age, no matter their income.

- The states and eligibility offers for Medicaid differ from state to state.

CHAPTER 4

Alzheimer's Diseases

~~~~~~~

Care with Love

Alois Alzheimer, a German psychiatrist, originally described Alzheimer's disease in 1906. Around 5.5 million Americans are living with Alzheimer's disease, making it the most common form of dementia in developed countries. Worldwide there are about 24 million people with Alzheimer's disease. Similarly, one in nine people over 65 has this disease and the likelihood of Alzheimer's increases with age.

Alzheimer's disease is a neurological condition that causes memory loss and cognitive decline. The disease usually begins slowly and gets worse over time. The brain structures most affected by Alzheimer's include the hippocampus (which controls memory), the amygdala (which helps regulate emotions), and the frontal cortex (which controls personality). As these areas deteriorate, a person feels more forgetfulness and changes in mood, behavior, or personality.

Alzheimer's disease causes memory loss, diminished ability to think clearly, and impaired judgment. However, it has no impact on a person's ability to feel or love. A person with this disease will still love you back just as much as they did before the diagnosis. Alzheimer's disease is not a normal part of aging, but as people live longer, they are prone to develop Alzheimer's or dementia at some point in their lives.

What causes Alzheimer's disease?

Many factors, including aging, genetics, head injuries, vascular disease, and infections linked to the cause of Alzheimer's disease. People with family members who have had Alzheimer's or dementia have a higher chance of developing it. Women are at greater risk than men because they live longer and tend to have higher estrogen levels in their bloodstreams after menopause — and estrogen has been linked to progressing Alzheimer's disease.

In addition, some studies suggest that certain lifestyle factors, such as obesity or lack of exercise, may increase your risk of developing Alzheimer's disease later on down the line. The first signs of Alzheimer's usually appear between the ages of 60 and 65 but can occur as early as age 30 or as late as 95. As the disease worsens, it becomes harder for a person to do day-to-day things and communicate with others.

SYMPTOMS

Alzheimer's disease can be hard for people to recognize in its early stages. These early signs include trouble following a conversation or remembering why a person just entered the room.

As the disease progresses, symptoms become more obvious and include:

- Problems with language and communication skills
- Changes in mood and personality
- Repetitive behaviors, such as talking continuously about unimportant matters.
- Asking the same question over and over again
- Disorientation with regard to time and place
- Difficulty carrying out routine activities.
- Difficulty identifying family members or friends who are close by.
- Trouble remembering recent events, names, or dates.
- Loss of balance when walking.
- Inability to sleep through the night

What are the different stages of Alzheimer's disease?

Alzheimer's is a progressive neurodegenerative disease affecting memory, language, and cognition. Four stages characterize it:

- Mild cognitive impairment (MCI)
- Mild Alzheimer's Disease (AD)
- Moderate AD
- Severe AD

The stages are based on how much function the patient can perform on their own and how well they can communicate with others. There is no known cure for Alzheimer's disease. Current treatments focus on addressing symptoms of the disease.

Mild Cognitive Impairment (MCI): Memory issues visible to others but does not significantly interfere with daily living.

Mild Alzheimer's Disease (AD): At this stage, symptoms become more severe and affect daily life significantly. People with mild AD can still recognize faces and remember things from their past well enough to live on their own, but they may have trouble remembering dates and times or doing complex tasks like learning new information or paying bills correctly.

Moderate Alzheimer's Disease (AD): People experience more severe cognitive problems such as confusion about time or place at this stage. In addition to their inability to identify family members or friends, they may also have problems speaking coherently or expressing themselves appropriately when interacting socially with others around them.

Severe dementia (AD): The last stage of Alzheimer's disease is called severe dementia. At this stage, the person with Alzheimer's has a loss of memory, communication skills, and function in daily activities. The person may become restless or agitated, have trouble sleeping and eating, and may need assistance with dressing, eating, and bathing.

What are the different types of Alzheimer's disease?

There are three types of Alzheimer's disease: Early Onset, Late Onset, and Mixed.

Early onset is uncommon, affects people under the age of 65, and accounts for less than 10% of all cases of the disease. It is caused by a change in the genes, which may cause memory loss to happen more quickly than in other types of Alzheimer's. Late Onset makes up 90% of cases, which occurs above 65 age. People with mixed Alzheimer's disease have early and late-onset Alzheimer's symptoms.

What to expect in different stages of Alzheimer's disease?

The primary stages of Alzheimer's are often labelled as Mild cognitive impairment or MCI. People with MCI who have no signs of dementia can live independently, but they may need more support than before they developed the condition. Individuals have trouble remembering names and dates or getting new information during this stage. They also have trouble finding words or focusing attention on a task.

In the middle stage of Alzheimer's, cognitive abilities will continue to decline, but it will gradually be difficult to recognize that there is an issue. Individuals will face difficulty completing familiar tasks and not recalling recent events well enough to talk about them with others. They also become confused when traveling from place to place and begin to lose interest in social activities like going out for dinner or visiting friends at home because it takes effort to stay focused on conversations with others around them.

What is the importance of having a caregiver when your loved one has Alzheimer's disease?

Alzheimer's patients need around-the-clock care because they have trouble communicating their needs or recognizing danger signals. You may not be able to provide this level of care independently, especially if you have other responsibilities like work or school. Almost 48% of nursing home residents suffer from Alzheimer's disease or other dementias. A professional caregiver can take over these tasks so that you can focus on what matters most: spending time with your loved one in the present moment.

The importance of having a caregiver when your loved one has Alzheimer's Disease is that they can help ease your loved one's stress and provide companionship, support, and assistance with day-to-day tasks. This can be especially important in the early stages of Alzheimer's when people are still capable of living independently but need help managing their day-to-day lives. This will make it easier for you to stay connected emotionally while still maintaining some independence in your life outside the home. In addition, having a caregiver around can give you peace of mind knowing that everything is being taken care of without worrying about whether there is enough food or medication available when needed or whether medications are being taken on time.

While there may be times when you feel like you're not able to give your loved one what they need due to factors like time constraints or personal health conditions (like fatigue), it's important to remember that there are many health care assistance options available to help you care for your loved one, such as nursing or assisted living homes.

How to care with love for someone with Alzheimer's disease?

It can be difficult to provide care for someone with Alzheimer's, but there are ways to help them feel loved even when they don't know who you are anymore. The first step is to determine what types of medications your loved one is taking and how they affect them. Many patients with Alzheimer's take medication that can make them more agitated or confused. You should then work with your loved one's doctor to develop a plan of action for dealing with those symptoms.

Even if you are not old or do not have a relative with Alzheimer's disease, being an "Alzheimer's caregiver" requires a great amount of patience. As the disease progresses, their behavior becomes even more unpredictable. A person with Alzheimer's has weaknesses in their memory, but it does not mean they have no feelings or emotions. Even if they cannot express their emotions well, they are still people who can be scared and confused.

While one day it might be possible to stop the progression of this disease and regenerate any lost brain cells, for the time being, there is no real treatment for Alzheimer's disease. Some caregivers have found that it helps to see their loved ones as still "there," even when they no longer recognize them. Music and TV are used as a way to draw their attention. This allows Alzheimer's patients to focus on something they used to enjoy, which can help them interact more easily with others. Caregivers who are struggling to readjust their thinking should know they are not alone; many people find this to be their most difficult challenge in caring for a loved one.

Next is to take special precautions and be aware of various safety issues when working with people with Alzheimer's. This can include helping the individual remain oriented, recognizing and addressing behavioral reactions, keeping your body movements slow and deliberate, and having a strategy for preventing accidents.

There are 3 main qualities to handling Alzheimer's patients: patience, support, and understanding. Here are ways to develop these qualities.

- Remind and express how you love them throughout the day by giving them hugs and kisses when appropriate.

- Show your love by playing music that reminds them of special moments between the two of you.

- Be patient and understanding. Remember that the person you are caring for is dealing with a huge amount of stress and confusion. They are probably frustrated and angry at times, but it is not their fault.

- Keep things simple and calm when possible. Try to keep your routine as normal as possible so that your loved ones can predict what might happen next—that way, they can feel more secure and less confused about what is going on around them!

- Keep their routine as consistent as possible while encouraging them to eat healthy meals at regular times each day.

- Approach the person gently and with sensitivity. Do not speak too loudly or angrily; do not show disappointment; always be sympathetic—but realistic.

- Make sure they get plenty of exercises each day or provide activities such as games or puzzles.

- Speak in simple words, using short sentences.

- Do not get frustrated with your loved ones if they forget something or do not understand what you are saying—remember that this is common for people with Alzheimer's disease.

- You can help by being aware of any changes in behavior and responding accordingly. For example, if your loved one is usually very calm but becomes agitated when you ask them to eat breakfast, try offering them a snack instead of making them sit at the table immediately.

- Treat their symptoms as best as you can. If they're having trouble remembering things or getting around on their own, then make sure you remind them of what time it is so they can plan ahead for appointments or important events like lunch dates with friends and family members; this will help reduce anxiety as well as increase independence.

How do you take care of yourself while caring for someone with Alzheimer's?

A survey by the Alzheimer's Association of both men and women found that 67% of caregivers who provide care for more than 21 hours are women. In addition, female caregivers have a higher strain, mood, depression, and health problems than male caregivers do because they tend to spend more time caring for someone with cognitive impairment. Hence, it is important at times to step back and reflect on how your mental health is affected by the act of caregiving.

Alzheimer's disease is a devastating, heartbreaking disease that knocks off people of their memories and personalities, but it does not have to rob you of all your life. The most important thing you can do is to care for yourself, so you can care for people with Alzheimer's disease. If you find yourself feeling exhausted, anxious, or overwhelmed, it may be time to take some steps toward self-care. Here are some ways:

- Make time for yourself: Take regular breaks from caring for others, even if they are only 5–10 minutes long. This will ensure that you are rested, calm, and prepared when it comes time to be there for your loved one again.

- Find support: Many online resources are designed specifically to help caregivers with Alzheimer's disease take care of themselves and their loved ones simultaneously. Check our website at [URL] or call us at [phone number]. We offer free consultations on how we can help ease your burden as a caregiver while maintaining.

- Assurance to yourself: Remember that it is okay — and normal — to feel frustrated sometimes. If you are under a lot of stress, it is perfectly normal to feel angry at times (just do not let those feelings build up inside until they turn into a rage). When these feelings arise, you might want to try journaling or to meditate instead of holding them in until they explode on someone else (such as a family member).

- Make sure to eat regular meals with healthy snacks in between, if necessary, so that you do not end up skipping meals because of stress or forgetfulness.

- Prioritize sleep. It is easy to lose track of time when caring for Alzheimer's patients and forget when it is time for bed or when you last ate.

Hence, make sure you set the alarm before going to bed at night and set the alarm on your phone during the day to remember when it is time for lunch or dinner.

The satisfaction of caring for people with Alzheimer's disease is priceless. It is a feeling that is deeply personal to each caregiver, and it is a feeling that they will never forget. You get to see the joy on their faces when they remember events from long ago; maybe it's a wedding they went to, a trip they took with their family, or even a favorite color. Whatever it is that brings joy to their lives — you are there to witness it. Most importantly, you get to be there for them in their time of need. The most important thing caregivers want is to feel like they are helping others; this is why so many people choose this path as a career.

"Too often we underestimate the power of a touch, a smile, a kind word, a listening ear, an honest compliment, or the smallest act of caring, all of which have the potential to turn a life around." – Leo Buscaglia

Key takeaway:

1. Alzheimer's disease affects around 5.5 million people in the United States.

2. Alzheimer's disease is characterized by a loss of memory, thinking, and reasoning skills.

3. The initial signs include behavioral changes, problems with communication, and forgetfulness.

4. Alzheimer's disease can affect anyone over 60 or as early as 30.

5. The 4 stages of Alzheimer's help understand how the disease progresses with time.

6. A professional caregiver caters to ensure they provide the support and medication needed for Alzheimer's patients.

7. The three main qualities of handling Alzheimer's patients are patience, support, and understanding.

8. The more you prioritize caring for your mental health, the easier it is to handle people with Alzheimer's disease.

CHAPTER 5

Dementia Disease

Care with Passion

Dementia is used to define a set of symptoms that can affect a person's capacity to perform everyday tasks. It is not a disease but a group of symptoms that affect an individual's behavior and lifestyle. Dementia affects an estimated 55 million people worldwide, with more than 60% living in developing countries. According to the United Nations, the number of people over the age of 65 will reach 78 million by 2030; with a 2:1 ratio, women are more likely to be affected than men.

Dementia occurs when brain cells called neurons die off at a faster rate than they are replaced, resulting in a build-up of plaques and tangles within the brain. These plaques and tangles interfere with normal brain function, causing symptoms such as confusion, forgetfulness, and difficulty finding words. Dementia can develop at any age after middle age but is frequently observed in people over 65 years old.

Alzheimer's disease causes approximately 60% of all dementia cases. Other types include Huntington's disease and Parkinson's disease, as well as vascular dementia (which develops after a stroke). In general, dementia means that your memory and thinking skills have become significantly impaired. You may have trouble remembering names or dates or struggle to focus on what you are reading. In severe cases, people with dementia are unable to communicate effectively and might get lost easily.

The first symptom of dementia is learning new information (retention) problems. As the condition progresses, people may lose their ability to remember recent events and may experience personality changes or mood swings. These symptoms are caused by disruption to neurons in the brain that make up certain regions responsible for memory processing.

What causes Dementia?

The causes of dementia can be due to genetics, lifestyle factors, and environmental factors such as pesticides and air pollution. Dementia can also occur as a result of medical conditions such as high blood pressure or diabetes. A doctor can tell if you have dementia by giving you a thorough exam and then testing for different kinds of dementia.

What are the signs of Dementia?

The signs of dementia can vary from one person to another. Some people with dementia may have difficulty remembering new information or abstract understanding concepts like humor or metaphors. Others may have problems with everyday tasks like paying bills, shopping for groceries, or navigating public transportation. These also include:

- Difficulty remembering recent events or conversations.

- Difficulty remembering words or understanding language.

- Problems with judgment and reasoning.

- Changes in personality or behavior.

What are the different types of Dementia?

There are many different types of dementia, and they can be further broken down into subtypes. The most common types of dementia include Alzheimer's disease, Vascular dementia, Lewy Body Dementia, Frontotemporal dementia, and Creutzfeldt-Jakob disease. People with dementia can develop these types when the symptoms worsen.

Alzheimer's disease accounts for 60–80% of dementia cases in older people. It is characterized by memory loss that worsens over time.

Vascular dementia is caused by a stroke or a series of mini-strokes in the brain. Vascular dementia occurs when blood vessels become damaged or blocked, leading to decreased oxygen flow to the brain. This type usually results in memory loss and difficulty with reasoning.

Lewy body dementia results from abnormal protein deposits within the brain that interfere with its structure and function. Lewy Body Dementia causes symptoms like those of Parkinson's disease — parkinsonian symptoms like tremors and slowness in movement — plus cognitive issues such as confusion and hallucinations; it tends to affect men more than women.

Frontotemporal Dementia: Affects the frontal lobes of the brain, causing emotional and behavioral problems as well as changes in speech patterns; it rarely affects memory or language skills. It can cause changes in personality, behavior, and memory loss.

Creutzfeldt - Jakob disease is caused by prions (infectious proteins) that attack brain cells; it can be passed on through contaminated surgical equipment.

What to expect in different stages of Dementia?

One of the most difficult parts of living with dementia is not being aware of what stage of the disease they are in and how it will progress. While every case of dementia progresses differently, knowing about the stages of dementia can help you better understand your loved one's symptoms and manage your care plan accordingly.

Dementia is a progressive condition in which the brain neutrons deteriorate and cannot function at their peak level. You can expect three stages of dementia: **Mild, Moderate, and Severe Dementia**.

1. Mild dementia involves memory loss that interferes with daily life but does not significantly interfere with the ability to perform work or other daily tasks. Early stage 1 is characterized by forgetting names for common objects or misplacing items within short distances. Though patients still recognize their memory deficit and feel distressed about it, they are able to compensate for it with less obvious means. Some individuals at this stage forget dates and specific events but can recall key points from long-term memory. However, deterioration happens quickly from here if not quickly treated.

2. Moderate dementia is characterized by reduced cognitive ability, such as difficulty remembering recent events or recognizing familiar people or places. The person may also have difficulties with language, communication, or problem-solving. However, the person can carry out basic self-care activities without assistance and live independently at home for most of the day. They might also know their own name and be able to give accurate details about their life history.

3. Severe dementia involves significant impairment of mental function that affects personal care skills (such as bathing and dressing), communication abilities (such as understanding spoken language), and/or social interactions with others (such as recognizing family members). At this stage, you will notice that your loved one no longer responds to normal verbal cues or attempts to have a conversation. They may ask you questions repeatedly or be confused about what time it is or where they are. They have difficulty remembering details of everyday life, such as meals, chores, errands, and appointments. It is important to note that even in the severe stage of Alzheimer's, you can still communicate with your loved one; they just may not always respond to your requests.

Importance of having a caregiver for people with Dementia

An estimated 11 million unpaid caregivers in the United States help people with Alzheimer's disease or another type of dementia. With almost 66% of caregivers living with a person with dementia in a community, it means you are more likely to come across a person with dementia through friends or family than with other diseases. According to the National Health and Wellness survey, the proportion of women caregivers in the United

States (61.5%) is higher than in European countries/regions (56.3%: France, Germany, the United Kingdom, Italy, and Spain).

A professional caregiver helps Alzheimer's patients with daily tasks and is also available for emotional support and companionship. They help keep your loved ones safe when you are present. They may not be able to remember things like where they need to go or what time it is, which could lead to them getting lost or at risk of injury if they do not have anyone around them. Hence, having someone to keep an eye on them can prevent these things from happening, so nothing goes wrong unexpectedly.

Studies have shown that proactive care for Alzheimer's and other dementias can significantly increase the quality of life for those who are affected and their caregivers. This step includes giving the best treatment options, participating in meaningful activities, learning more about the disease, or even connecting with a support group. A caregiver that cares passionately for people with dementia finds gratitude and strength in the process.

How to care with a passion for someone with Dementia?

Caring for someone with dementia can be quite difficult, both for the person who has it and their loved ones. It can be easy to feel overwhelmed by your loved one's forgetfulness, mood swings, and other aspects of the disease. As the symptoms of dementia worsen, caregivers can experience emotional stress, depression, and health problems. Remember that you are not obliged to control other people's situations but can control how you react to them. The best way to honor those who suffer from this terrible disease is by facing it with optimism and strength. There are ways to care for someone with dementia that can help them feel more comfortable and safe.

First, it is important to remember that dementia affects everyone differently. What works for one person may not work for another. Therefore, you need to be flexible in how you approach the situation. Some people with dementia like having a routine. They may benefit from knowing exactly what time they are going to eat, sleep, or do other activities during the day. Other people with dementia may prefer less structure in their days—they may appreciate scheduled activities but not necessarily have a set time when those activities will happen each day. You must try different things out until you find what works best for your loved one's needs and personality type, so they feel happy and comfortable in their current situation.

Here are some tips to keep in mind when caring for someone with dementia:

- Be mindful of their feelings. If something makes them uncomfortable or unhappy, stop immediately.

- Make sure they have something to do while you are busy with other things, like reading a book or watching TV together.

- Let them know what's happening around them, so they don't feel like they're being left out or forgotten about (even if it's just something small like mentioning what color shirt you're wearing today).

- Avoid arguments: Arguing with a person with dementia, especially with an episode, will only frustrate them and make matters worse. Try not to take their words or actions personally; do your best to understand that you are dealing with a person who is experiencing many physical and mental issues. You may want to use gestures or a calming tone of voice instead of talking at them.

How to Maintain Your Sanity While Caring for a Loved One with Dementia

Dementia is an unfortunate part of aging and devastating to the entire family. It can strain relationships and tear families apart, causing them to question why they should even bother to take care of their loved ones if they cannot remember them anyway. Nevertheless, you owe it to your parents, spouse, siblings, or friends to do everything you can to care for them as best you can—and that includes taking care of yourself along the way. According to a study published in 2019, the average time spent by informal caregivers of people with dementia is 5 hours per day. This can be overwhelming, both physically and emotionally, as well as financially.

Getting caught up in the stress of caring for someone who needs extra attention is easy. However, if you do not take care of yourself, you will burn out and be unable to provide the best care possible. Here are some tips for taking care of yourself while caring for someone with dementia:

- Stay active: You need physical activity to stay healthy, but exercising too much can make you tired or sore. Make sure you only do activities you enjoy because they give you energy instead of making you feel tired afterward.

- Make sure to eat regular meals, even if your loved one is not eating much. You need to have enough energy to provide the best care possible.

- Try not to stress out about things beyond your control that may be causing problems with your loved one's health or behavior (such as medications that are not working right).

- Get support from friends and family members who understand what you are going through. It is important to be able to talk about what you are feeling without hiding it away—it will help you feel less isolated and more connected with those around you who can relate to your situation.

"The disease might hide the person underneath, but there's still a person in there who needs your love and attention." — Jamie Calandriello

Key Takeaways:

- An estimated 55 million people worldwide suffer from dementia, and people over the age of 65 will reach 78 million by 2030.

- Dementia occurs when brain cells called neurons die off at a faster rate than they are replaced.

- Alzheimer's disease accounts for 60% of dementia cases.

- The first symptoms of dementia are problems with learning new information and recalling events.

- The causes of dementia can be due to genetics, lifestyle factors, and environmental factors such as pesticides and air pollution.

- There are three stages of dementia— Mild, Moderate, and Severe Dementia.

- It is necessary to have a caregiver look over a person with severe or moderate dementia.

- To care for people with dementia includes having traits of optimism and strength, despite not remembering you.

CHAPTER 6

Parkinson's Disease

~~~~~

Care With Positivity

In 1817, James Parkinson recorded the first case of Parkinson's disease in a 50-year-old man with tremors, slow movement, and rigidity. His essay described this disease as "shaking palsy" due to its early physical symptoms. Parkinson's disease is a chronic condition that affects the area of the brain responsible for movement. Parkinson's disease is caused by a lack of dopamine, a neurotransmitter (signalling molecule) that controls muscle movements and coordination. The loss of these cells leads to a decrease in dopamine production, which causes problems with movement and balance. It is characterized by tremors and a loss of muscle control.

According to the Parkinson's Foundation, 10 million people live with Parkinson's disease worldwide. Of those, 1 million people come from the United States alone, and about 60,000 Americans are diagnosed annually. Parkinson's disease develops under older age. However, only 4% of people are diagnosed before 50. Men are 1.5 times more likely to develop the disease than women.

People with Parkinson's disease feel like they are in a constant state of falling. They cannot make their bodies do what they want them to do, and they feel like they are out of control. Some people experience this as a feeling of "being disconnected" from their bodies, while others experience it as a feeling of being stuck in their bodies. This can be mild and manageable in the primary stages of the disease. However, as the disease progresses, it can become more and more difficult to do basic things like walking or picking up objects.

What causes Parkinson's disease?

A 2018 journal research on the environmental factors found several risk factors linked to Parkinson's disease, including smoking, consuming coffee, engaging in strenuous activity, taking ibuprofen, having high plasma urate levels, using certain pesticides, and suffering a traumatic brain injury. Most people who get Parkinson's disease do not get it directly from their families. Instead, they get it from a complex mix of genetic and environmental factors.

What are the signs of Parkinson's disease?

The common early symptom of Parkinson's disease is tremors. Tremors in the hands and feet are the most common primary signs of Parkinson's disease. Other symptoms include subtle changes in behaviour or mood. These include:

- Depression
- Anxiety
- Social withdrawal
- Changes in sleep patterns
- Loss of sense of smell or taste (usually mild)
- Constipation (usually mild)
- Urinary difficulties (difficulty starting urination, weak stream, dribbling after urinating)
- Stiffness - slow movements and stiffness in the neck, arms, or legs that are difficult to relax.
- The rigidity-muscle tone that is hard to move
- Bradykinesia - slowness, and difficulty in initiating movement, may also experience difficulty swallowing or chewing food due to slow movement of muscles needed for these activities.
- Postural instability - problems standing up from sitting or lying down

As the disorder progresses, these symptoms may become more severe to the point where they interfere with daily activities like walking or eating. As the disease progresses, it can cause speech difficulties, depression, dementia, and other cognitive issues.

What are the different types of Parkinson's disease?

According to the Parkinson's Foundation, approximately 15% of people with PD have one of several disorders called "atypical parkinsonism disorders". These conditions are more difficult to treat than PD, and the types include:

Multiple System Atrophy (MSA): Multiple system atrophy (MSA) is a group of neurodegenerative disorders characterized by the deterioration of several different body systems (neurological, autonomic, and musculoskeletal). MSA causes people to move slowly and lose their balance. They also have trouble controlling their blood pressure and bladders.

Progressive Supranuclear Palsy (PSP): Patients with PSP have difficulty moving their eyes up and down, which can lead to falls. These patients also have problems swallowing, speaking, sleeping, remembering, and thinking clearly. This disease usually develops in the mid-40s.

Corticobasal Syndrome (CBS): CBS is a rare form of Parkinson's disease that typically begins after age 60 and initially affects a limb. Other symptoms can include involuntary jerking movements (myoclonus), difficulty with certain motor tasks despite normal muscle strength (apraxia), and trouble understanding language (aphasia).

What are the different stages of Parkinson's disease?

Parkinson's disease is a neurological disorder that affects movement actions. It is caused by the loss of dopamine-producing brain cells, which leads to tremors, stiffness, and muscle weakness.

There are four main types of Parkinson's disease:

1) Early Onset PD - People with early onset PD typically develop symptoms between the ages of 30 and 60 years old. They may also have trouble sleeping or feeling restless.

2) Late-onset PD - People with late-onset PD typically develop symptoms after age 60. The person with Parkinson's may start to have difficulty walking or doing simple tasks like buttoning their shirt or turning off a light switch. As the disease advances even further, it can lead to cognitive impairment (memory loss). This is because dopamine levels drop rapidly at this stage—which is why it's called "dopamine depletion" or "dopaminergic deficiency"—and this leads to problems with thinking clearly and not remembering things clearly.

3) Autosomal Dominant PD - This type of PD occurs when one parent has the disease and passes on the genetic mutation to their child. This type of PD accounts for 5-10% of all cases of Parkinson's disease.

4) Sporadic PD -Sporadic PD accounts for 90–95% of all cases of Parkinson's disease, meaning that it occurs randomly in people with no family history or genetic links to the condition.

What is the importance of having a caregiver when your loved one has Parkinson's disease?

If you are caring for someone with Parkinson's disease, then you know how difficult it can be to manage all of the symptoms associated with this illness. The tremors, rigidity, and loss of mobility can make it hard to get around and do everyday tasks like going to work or taking care of household chores. People with Parkinson's often need help from their caregivers to be able to do things. An experienced home care assistant can keep them from feeling helpless and alone.

When your loved one has Parkinson's disease, you may be tempted to try to do everything yourself. After all, they are your family—of course, you want to help and support them through this difficult time. Unfortunately, Parkinson's disease is progressive and will worsen over time. Your loved one will need more assistance as time goes on. That is where a caregiver comes in. A caregiver can assist with daily living activities such as eating and dressing or help with transportation and preparing meals for your loved one. They can also help keep track of medications and other parts of care that need to be looked after on a regular basis.

People living with PD often experience loneliness, as they cannot do all the things they used to enjoy doing because of their condition. Having someone there who listens to them talk about their day or spends time together doing nothing can improve their quality of life.

The Power of Positivity: How to Care for Someone with Parkinson's disease

Parkinson's disease affects millions of people around the world, but that does not mean it has to be a negative experience. With a positive attitude, care, and support from friends and family, life can still be as fulfilling as possible. Parkinson's disease can be managed through medication, physical therapy, and lifestyle changes such as exercise and diet. Caring for someone with Parkinson's requires patience, compassion, and understanding of what the person needs and wants. Here are some tips on how to care with positivity for someone with Parkinson's disease:

- Be aware of any particular triggers that may upset your loved one, such as loud noises or bright lights.

- Make sure your loved one has access to all their medications and medical supplies in one place, so they do not have trouble finding what they need when they need it.

- Help them set up an alert system for when they are alone in case something happens. This can include a phone call or text message.

- • Try not to over-react when they do something that might seem unusual or strange because of their Parkinson's disease (e.g., walking hunched over or having trouble writing down notes).

- Try not to make jokes about their condition; it will hurt their feelings and may cause them to withdraw from you.

- Make sure your home is safe for someone with Parkinson's disease. Consider installing handrails in the bathroom and a nightlight in the hallways, so it is easier for them to get around at night.

- Encourage them to take daily walks outside if possible — even if they only walk around the block once per day. Even if it's just a few minutes each day, this can help improve balance and coordination as well as reduce depression, which often occurs with Parkinson's disease due to anxiety caused by disability or loss of independence.

How to take care of yourself while caring for someone with Parkinson's disease?

Caring for a person with Parkinson's disease can be emotionally and physically challenging. Stress and depression can make it harder to care for your loved one making it harder for you to take care of yourself. As Parkinson's disease progresses, caregivers experience fatigue and excessive daytime sleepiness that interferes with their daily lives. This can cause frustration to caregivers, who provide more hands-on assistance as the immobility increases. Caring for someone else is an incredibly stressful job, and you need to be able to make time for yourself so that you stay healthy enough to do it well. Here are some tips:

- If your loved one has trouble sleeping, consider setting up his room with a white noise machine or fan. This can help mask noise from outside the room and make sleeping easier for your loved one.

- Consider getting a massage or a pedicure as a treat for yourself when you need it most.

- Maintain a healthy diet by eating healthy foods and staying hydrated throughout the day—you will feel better if you take care of yourself along with your loved ones.

- Do not isolate yourself from friends and family— hang out with other people, so you do not feel alone or overwhelmed by what is happening at home.

"Caregiving often calls us to lean into love we didn't know possible." — *Tia Walker*

Key takeaways:

- Ten million people worldwide live with Parkinson's disease; men are more likely to develop it.

- Parkinson's disease affects the region of the brain responsible for movement regulation.

- The cause of Parkinson's disease can be due to environmental and genetic factors.

- Signs of Parkinson's disease include the constant movement of specific body parts and changes in behaviour, mood, or posture.

- Parkinson's disease is a progressive disorder that will worsen over time.

- Caring for Parkinson's disease patients includes being compassionate and optimistic despite their situation.

- Parkinson's disease can be managed through constant medication, physical therapy, and better lifestyle choices.

- Keeping your mental health in check is crucial to best care for someone with Parkinson's disease.

CHAPTER 7

Osteoporosis Disease

～～

Care With Smile

Osteoporosis is a disease in which the bones become weak and brittle and easily fracture. It occurs when the body does not produce new bone or does not maintain old bone, leading to a loss in bone mass. This can cause the bones to break effortlessly, resulting in pain and disability. This condition typically affects older people, and women are more likely to develop it than men. The most common areas of fracture are the spine, wrist, and hip. A person with osteoporosis experiences pain when standing or walking, limping, back pain, and difficulty sleeping.

Osteoporosis affects an estimated 200 million individuals worldwide. According to the International Osteoporosis Foundation's statistics, one in five women over the age of 50 and one in five men suffer an osteoporotic fracture at some point in their lives. Osteoporosis affects an estimated 10 million people in the United States aged 50 and over. While over 43 million additional adults have poor bone mass, they are likely to develop osteoporosis.

Osteoporosis is treatable if the condition is diagnosed at an early stage with medication and lifestyle changes. If left untreated, osteoporosis can cause serious health problems like unhealed broken bones and prevent mobility. Therefore, caregivers and family members should learn about the disease to keep patients from getting hurt in the future.

What causes Osteoporosis Disease?

The most common cause of osteoporosis is age-related bone loss (known as senile osteoporosis), which occurs in most people after age 50. However, osteoporosis can occur at any age and is more common in women after menopause. Other causes of osteoporosis include: not getting enough calcium or vitamin D; smoking; long-term use of corticosteroids; excessive alcohol intake; being overweight or underweight; having a family history of osteoporosis; taking medications such as certain anti-seizure drugs or cancer chemotherapy medicines that affect bone health, and having certain medical conditions such as hyperparathyroidism (overactive parathyroid gland) or Cushing's syndrome (excessive secretion of cortisol).

What are the signs of Osteoporosis Disease?

The most common sign of osteoporosis is broken bones. Other signs include:

- Sudden fractures occur from a minor fall or bump into something.

- Pain in your back and spine when moving around.

- Back pain, spine pain, joint pain, joint stiffness, dizziness, or balance problems.

- Loss of height due to vertebrae collapsing inwardly (this can lead to stooped posture).

- Achy pain in fingers or toes when grabbing something tightly.

- Feeling tired than usual

What are the different types of Osteoporosis Disease?

There are two main types of osteoporosis: **Primary osteoporosis** and **Secondary osteoporosis.**

- Primary osteoporosis occurs when the body's healthy new bone tissue production slows down, resulting in thinning bones. The bones begin to lose density and strength due to age, genetics, or lifestyle factors.

- Secondary osteoporosis occurs when there is an underlying condition that causes bone loss. This can include kidney failure, lung disease, cancer, rheumatoid arthritis, or other conditions.

The two types of osteoporosis are treated differently. For example, primary osteoporosis may require therapy or medications to help stimulate bone building, while secondary osteoporosis will require additional treatment for the original condition causing bone loss.

What are the different stages of Osteoporosis Disease?

Worldwide, osteoporosis causes more than 8.9 million fractures annually. Hence, it is important to be aware of these stages to help patients get early treatment to prevent further damage.

- The first stage of osteoporosis is called pre-osteoporosis. The bone mineral density is significantly lower than normal, but it is not at the level required to diagnose osteoporosis.

- The second stage of the disease is called "osteopenia." It is when the bones have started to become thinner, but they have not yet broken down. The bones have low bone mass but are still strong enough to support the body. There is no treatment at this stage unless the fracture risk is high. The patient needs to continue exercising and eating healthy foods to help strengthen their bones.

- The third stage of osteoporosis is known as severe osteoporosis. At this stage, 30% of bone mass is lost, and at high risk of fractures, deformities, joint pain, etc.

During each stage of the disease, individuals are at a higher risk of bone fractures due to weak bones, which can easily break under stress or pressure.

What is the importance of having a caregiver when your loved one has Osteoporosis Disease?

Osteoporosis can be treated with medications and changes in lifestyle such as exercise, weight control, smoking cessation, and reduction of alcohol consumption. However, there are many instances where this condition does not respond well to these measures or when there are other underlying health conditions. In these cases, patients must have some form of assistance with their daily activities, such as grocery shopping and cleaning.

Having an extra hand can help your loved one remain independent in their home and avoid moving into health care facilities. In addition, it can help family members get a break from being the primary caretaker and their day-to-day responsibilities.

How to care with a smile for someone with Osteoporosis Disease?

Osteoporosis disease tends to be a silent killer. That is because, while a healthy adult may only break a bone or two in his life, those with osteoporosis often break bones several times a year. They are ten times more likely to fracture their spine than the average person. Patients with osteoporosis disease need encouragement to maintain their mental and physical abilities. They can feel like a burden if not treated with gestures of open hearts. Here are some tips to get started:

Encourage to Exercise: Exercising helps strengthen muscles and bones, which can make bones stronger. Ask your loved one if they would like to try walking, light swimming, or dancing. If they are not interested in exercising yet, you should encourage them to do so anyway because it will help them stay healthy as they age. For patients with kyphosis and back pain, weight-bearing exercises, back strengthening, and balance training can improve their gait.

Careful with falls: If someone with osteoporosis falls, it could cause serious injury or even death. They might also break their bones if they fall while walking or climbing stairs. To help prevent falls, create safe pathways in your home and keep clutter out of common areas like kitchens or bathrooms so that people do not trip over things when moving around the house. You can also help by making sure that household appliances have non-skid pads underneath them so that if someone does slip on them, there will not be any serious injuries.

Nutritious Diet: Make sure your loved one gets enough calcium each day by giving them plenty of milk or cheese products. As a caregiver, you can encourage them to eat healthy foods by stocking up on fruits and vegetables and offering these items first when preparing meals for yourself or others in your household. You should also encourage your loved one to avoid eating too much salt or sugar because these can cause dehydration, which can lead to bone loss over time if left untreated. While all foods contain some nutrients, some foods are particularly high in calcium and vitamin D. These include:

- Milk and dairy products such as cheese and yogurt
- Salmon (wild-caught)
- Kale and spinach (cooked)
- Dark leafy greens like collard greens and kale

Fractures caused by Osteoporosis can be painful and debilitating, not to mention harmful to an older body. People with Osteoporosis can move around safely and independently by taking steps to prevent falls.

How to take care of yourself while caring for someone with Osteoporosis Disease?

Caring for them at home can be challenging if you or someone you love has been diagnosed with osteoporosis disease. How do you take care of your daily tasks, including cooking and cleaning, while providing the 24/7 assistance needed by someone with osteoporosis? The key to taking care of yourself and your loved one at the same time is to plan ahead before an emergency happens so that you can remain calm during those times of crisis. Here are the top five ways to take care of yourself while caring for someone with osteoporosis disease in the home.

- Make time for yourself. This means taking breaks when necessary and not feeling guilty about them. It also means ensuring that your needs as an individual are met — not just the needs of your loved one. If you are having trouble remembering this, consider keeping a journal where you can write down things that have been stressful lately or things that make you happy so that they are always in sight.

- Setting boundaries between your personal and professional lives can help you stay focused on what really matters. You will feel more relaxed about your work and can do both jobs better when you know where the line is drawn between them. Setting boundaries also means being clear about how much time you are taking away from yourself for work and how much time you are giving back.

- Get plenty of rest. Resting helps keep muscles healthy and strong.

- Do not let negative thoughts rule you. If you find yourself dwelling on negative thoughts and emotions that stop you from getting out of bed or from going to work, seek professional help.

The best course of action is to think of self-management as a lifelong commitment. It is important to remain proactive in the maintenance of your health and learn about osteoporosis at every stage of a patient's life so you can provide them with the necessary care throughout their journey.

"Be helpful. When you see a person without a smile, give them yours." — *Zig Ziglar*

Key takeaway:

- Osteoporosis is a disease that causes bones to become thinner and weaker. It is common in older people but can affect anyone at any age.

- Women tend to develop osteoporosis disease more than men.

- The primary cause of osteoporosis is age-related bone loss, which occurs in most people after age 50.

- Being aware of the three stages can help patients get early treatment to prevent further damage.

- Osteoporosis can be treated with medications and lifestyle changes such as exercise, weight control, smoking cessation, and reduction of alcohol consumption.

CHAPTER 8

Chronic Kidney Disease

≈≋≋≋≋

Care With Attention

Chronic disease is a progressive condition in which the kidneys lose their ability to filter toxins and waste products from the blood. The kidneys are responsible for removing waste products from the blood, including urea, creatinine, and other substances. Therefore, the kidneys are vital to the proper functioning of the body.

In most cases, chronic kidney disease is caused by diabetes. In these cases, fatty deposits called atherosclerotic plaques clog the blood vessels that supply and drain blood flow to and from the kidneys. These deposits are made up of cholesterol, cellular debris, fat, and other proteins. When there is plenty of plaque in the arteries leading to the kidneys, it clogs them and prevents them from working properly. In the worst cases, dialysis or a transplant becomes necessary to survive.

It is estimated that around 840 million people worldwide are affected by chronic kidney disease. In the U.S. alone, 15% of adults have the disease, although most only find out about it in the later stages.

What causes chronic kidney disease?

Chronic kidney disease is a condition that affects a person's ability to retain fluid. The primary cause of chronic kidney disease is hypertension, which increases the pressure in the arteries that feed blood to the kidneys. This causes damage to these organs and impairs their ability to filter blood properly.

Other factors associated with chronic kidney disease include high blood levels of lipids (fats), proteins, and glucose that can result from high cholesterol levels; high blood pressure; obesity; diabetes; and high salt intake. In people with diabetes, their bodies are unable to use insulin efficiently. Because of this, too much sugar builds up in the blood and can damage the kidneys.

What are the signs of chronic kidney disease?

Chronic kidney disease may not cause symptoms until years after it has begun to take hold. If you have chronic kidney disease, you may always find yourself tired with no energy to do anything productive. You may also notice your skin starting to break out with pimples or developing dark patches on your face that do not go away with lotion. These symptoms can be mistaken for aging as they occur gradually over time—chronic kidney disease is not something you can catch overnight. Some of the most common symptoms include:

- Anemia (low red blood cell counts)

- Back pain or stiffness
- Unexpected weight loss, changes in appetite or thirst
- Confusion or memory problems related to confusion or memory problems related to dementia.
- Recurring fever and chills
- Urine output that is low or non-existent
- Urine with dark-colored or turbid sediment
- Urinary tract infections (UTIs)
- Difficulty urinating due to pain or pressure in the lower abdomen or back
- Jaundice (yellowing of the skin and eyes)
- Frequent urination

What are the different types of chronic kidney disease?

There are several different types of chronic kidney disease (CKD). These include:

Chronic Kidney Disease of Unknown Origin (CKDUO): This is one of the most common kidney diseases, characterized by the absence of symptoms or changes in kidney function. It can develop over time and lead to a high risk of further complications, including cardiovascular disease, diabetes, and hypertension.

Post-transplant chronic kidney disease: After receiving a new kidney transplant, some people will develop post-transplant CKD that lasts for months or years after they receive their new organ. This type of CKD is treated with medications or dietary changes.

Kidney stones: Stones can form in either one or both kidneys. However, they do not usually cause any symptoms until they become large enough to block urine flow from one side of the body into another.

End-Stage Renal Disease (ESRD): This is a more advanced form of CKD where your kidneys have failed to function effectively, and you need dialysis or other medical treatment to survive.

Diabetic Nephropathy: It develops when you have diabetes and high blood pressure. It causes damage to your kidneys over time but does not affect their ability to filter waste products from your blood as ESRD does.

Polycystic kidney disease: This illness causes cysts to form in the kidneys, which can eventually cause the kidneys to fail.

Kidney infection (Pyelonephritis): An inflammation of the kidneys is caused by a bacterial or viral infection. It occurs in people with diabetes mellitus (severely high blood sugar) or may happen after a kidney transplant.

Glomerulonephritis is an inflammation of the glomeruli—the tiny blood vessels inside the kidney

that filter blood before it enters the body. This happens when there is damage to these tiny blood vessels, usually because of a blockage or infection.

End-stage renal disease (ESRD): This is the final stage of chronic kidney disease where the kidneys can no longer function. The treatment options range from dialysis and transplantation to a combination of dialysis and transplantation.

What to expect in different stages of chronic kidney disease?

The different stages of chronic kidney disease are:

1. **Pre-clinical stage:** This stage is characterized by normal kidney function. At this stage, the patient may still be able to work and perform some activities without any problems.

2. **Mild-stage CKD:** At this stage, the kidney function gradually reduces, which causes an increase in the risk for complications. The patient can still manage their life without too many problems. However, the patient should be closely monitored at this stage to ensure that there are no complications arising from CKD. Mild-stage CKD patients may experience symptoms like fatigue, muscle cramps, nausea, weight loss, and other symptoms related to fluid retention. They

do not have any significant health issues such as high blood pressure or diabetes yet.

3. **Moderate-stage CKD:** This stage is characterized by moderately reduced kidney function that causes an increased risk for complications. Symptoms such as nausea and vomiting or a loss of appetite are common. The patient will experience some limitations in their daily activities due to their lower kidney function, such as difficulty urinating or passing blood in stools or urine more often than usual during a given time period (known as hematuria).

4. **Severe-stage CKD:** This stage is characterized by severely reduced kidney function that leads to end-stage kidney failure (kidney failure). At this point, it becomes important for doctors and family members to find out if a suitable donor organ is available so they can remain alive long enough to receive one or to put the patient under dialysis.

What is the importance of having a caregiver when your loved one has chronic kidney disease?

Having a caregiver can make all the difference for someone with chronic kidney disease, as they may require dialysis three times a week. In order to do this, they will need a caregiver who can take them to the dialysis center and then stay with them until they have finished their treatment. Having caregivers is crucial because it allows your loved ones to remain in their own homes and continue living as normally as possible.

Caregiving can give support with daily activities such as cooking, cleaning, shopping, and other maintenance tasks that they may not be able to do by themselves due to their illness. Having a caregiver can also help you feel more confident about being able to care for your loved one because you will know that someone is there for them if something goes wrong or if there are any changes in their health status. They can live at home longer if they have someone else around who cares for them around the clock.

It will also give them someone they can confide in about their condition and its effects on their health, so they know they're not alone in feeling helpless. Having someone who understands what it feels like to live with a similar condition will make it easier to manage their symptoms and create positive changes in their lifestyle.

People with this disease have kidneys that no longer work properly to filter waste out of their blood. This causes high levels of waste in the blood and makes it hard to stay hydrated or healthy. Hence, having someone around who will help make sure you are getting enough fluids and nutrients through food or drink, as well as help with medications, can significantly improve their lives.

How do you take care of and pay attention to someone with chronic kidney disease?

When monitored properly, chronic kidney disease can be managed through dietary changes and medication so that patients can maintain a quality of life as long as possible. Several lifestyle factors can increase your risk of chronic kidney disease, including high blood pressure, diabetes, and obesity. However, you can decrease your risk by controlling these factors with the following tips on caring for someone with chronic kidney disease.

It's also important for people with chronic kidney disease to eat well and get enough rest so that they're not feeling too tired all the time. This also includes:

- Limit alcohol consumption or smoking because these things can make their kidneys work harder than normal, leading to even more damage over time.

- Do not worry if someone with chronic kidney disease does not eat much or drink much water. It is normal for someone with chronic kidney disease to feel thirsty and needs more fluids than usual.

- Be sure to get regular checkups with the doctor or nurse practitioner to monitor any changes in symptoms or health status over time since the diagnosis was made (or even before). This will allow you to ensure everything is going well and there are no complications from their disease process.

- Make sure you have access to the supplies they need on hand. This includes pain medication, antibiotics, and other medications or supplements.

- Give them time for enough rest. Chronic kidney disease is exhausting, so if they are not feeling well, make sure that they get plenty of sleep and don't feel like they have an obligation to take care of themselves.

Chronic kidney disease has a high risk of high blood pressure. High blood pressure can damage the kidneys and lead to kidney failure. There are several steps to lower blood pressure and prevent kidney disease:

- Aim for a healthy weight. Excess weight is a major factor in high blood pressure.

- Control sodium intake by consuming fewer processed foods and more fresh fruits, vegetables, lean meats, whole grains, low-fat dairy products, and fish.

- Get regular exercise for the heart rate to stay steady.

How to take care of yourself while caring for someone with chronic kidney disease?

You cannot care for someone properly if you are neglecting your own needs. It is also important to remember that you are not alone in this journey: many people have gone through similar experiences, and there are many resources out there for both caregivers and those who need care. Here are some tips to help you stay healthy and happy while taking care of someone with chronic kidney disease:

- Be patient and kind to yourself. Do not beat yourself up when you feel down or anxious. It is perfectly normal to have bad days or weeks at times.

- Share what you are going through with others who have been there before. Talking about your feelings helps others understand what you are going through and may provide some relief in the process.

- Take care of your own mental health first by finding healthy coping mechanisms and setting boundaries that help you feel safe and secure at the moment.

- If you care for someone, avoid taking on their feelings or responses as your own—it can be difficult to distinguish between being empathetic and getting overwhelmed by your emotions. Remember that your patient may not be able to express what is happening inside them, so let them tell you when they need some space or just want someone else to talk with them about something else.

Key takeaways:

- Chronic disease is a progressive condition that causes the kidneys to lose their ability to filter toxins and waste products from the blood.

- The initial sign of chronic illness is when the body lacks the energy to do anything or signs of skin patches.

- There are several types of chronic diseases, each with its own symptoms.

- Caregiving for chronic disease patients is important to help them cope, as the condition can lead to several complications, including fatigue and fluid retention.

- It can be easy to get so caught up in taking care of your loved one that you forget to take care of yourself, but it's important to remember that you can't be your best self if you're not taking care of your own health.

CHAPTER 9

Stroke

~~~~~~~~

Care And Advocate For Your Loved One

A stroke is a medical condition in which blood that flows to part of the brain is interrupted or disrupted. This blockage can be caused by a blood clot, an aneurysm, or an abnormal accumulation of blood pressure inside an artery. It is an interruption in the blood supply to part of the brain, which deprives that part of oxygen and glucose. The deprivation causes cell death or damage to those cells that impact the respective organ. The part of the brain affected by a stroke can range from one region to another, and the severity of the symptoms depends on where in the brain they occur.

Stroke is the second leading cause of death. Every year, 15 million people all over the world suffer from a stroke. Over 1 in 4 people in the U.S. have a record of getting a stroke, in which the majority of strokes are ischemic strokes. Although it is unclear why some people are more susceptible to certain types of strokes than others, there are some risk factors to be aware of. These include:

- **Age:** A person's risk of having a stroke increases as they get older.

- **Gender:** Women tend to have more strokes than men do, but that may be because women are more likely to die from heart disease and other causes before they develop strokes.

- **Race/Ethnicity:** People who are African American or Hispanic have a higher risk of suffering a stroke than other racial groups.

What causes a stroke?

Strokes are most common among people over 65 and those with high blood pressure (hypertension), smoking, diabetes, and high cholesterol levels. High blood pressure, smoking, high cholesterol levels, diabetes, obesity, and certain heart problems cause strokes.

In some cases, vascular diseases, which are also called "hardening of the arteries," cause strokes. Other diseases like atherosclerosis cause plaque buildup on the inner walls of arteries. This plaque then thins out over time and weakens the wall of the artery until there's no more support for it. This results in a blockage that can lead to a stroke.

What are the signs of a stroke?

The first sign of a stroke is a sudden onset of numbness or weakness in the arms and legs, followed by blurred vision, slurred speech, and difficulty swallowing. If the person experiences weakness on one side of their body, numbness, and altered sensations in their face or arms, they are likely to experience a stroke.

The signs of a stroke are:

- Sudden numbness or weakness in the face, arm, or leg.
- Sudden confusion, trouble speaking or understanding speech, or loss of balance or coordination.
- Sudden trouble seeing in one or both eyes.
- Sudden trouble walking, dizziness, loss of balance or coordination suddenly.

In some cases, there may be no symptoms until several hours after the stroke. In these cases, it is important to call emergency services immediately if the person experiences any of the above signs of a stroke.

What are the different types of strokes?

There are five different kinds of stroke:

1. **Ischemic stroke** accounts for 80% of all strokes and can occur when there are blockages in arteries around your heart or neck veins. A piece of debris (like a clump of fatty tissue) breaks off from another area and travels through your bloodstream toward the heart. These are usually

mild and may happen when you have an episode of dizziness or a headache that lasts for less than 24 hours.

2. **Intracerebral hemorrhage:** The second most common stroke is caused by bleeding between two layers of tissue inside the skull (the meninges) due to trauma such as a fall or head injury, infection, or inheritance.

3. **Thromboembolism** refers to any obstruction in one or more arteries leading up to the heart. It can be caused by atherosclerosis (hardening/clogging of your arteries), heart disease (such as angina pectoris), or other conditions (such as having had recent surgery).

4. **Hemorrhagic stroke** occurs when blood vessels in the brain burst, leaking blood into the surrounding tissue. This causes damage to cells and tissue, which results in loss of function and permanent disability or death. The symptoms include confusion and loss of consciousness, which can last from hours to days depending on how severe it is.

5. **Cerebrovascular accident (CVA):** A CVA is caused by a blockage in an artery that supplies blood to the brain or spinal cord. Dizziness, numbness, weakness, and trouble speaking,

writing or processing words are among the symptoms.

What are the different stages of a stroke?

A person with a stroke will go through five stages of recovery. It is important to know your patient's stages.

The first stage is **flaccidity**. This is when the brain is not functioning properly and has lost its ability to control muscles.

The second stage is **spasticity**. At this stage, the person's muscles are overactive or underactive, depending on how much they are affected by the stroke. Spasticity can cause pain and difficulty in walking or standing up. It can also affect breathing and blood circulation.

The third stage is **complex movement combinations** in which the person is not able to move independently of one side of their body. This occurs because of damage to one side of the brain.

The fourth stage is **spasticity disappearing**, and the fifth and final stage is a normal function returning; this usually occurs within three to four hours after the onset of symptoms.

What is the importance of having a caregiver when your loved one has a stroke?

While most strokes are treated with medication, some people will require long-term care after they have been discharged from the hospital. The patient's family may choose to hire a home health aide, or personal care worker (PCP), who can help with personal care such as bathing and feeding, dressing, toileting, and transferring from a wheelchair to bed.

The significance of having caregivers is determined by several factors, including how much independence your loved one had prior to their stroke. Is he/she able to get around on their own? Do you want someone who will stay with them 24 hours a day? Or do you prefer an overnight house sitter? These are all important questions when choosing a caregiver for your loved one after a stroke.

By having someone in their lives who understands what type of care they need and how to provide it, they can live independently with fewer restrictions on their activities.

In addition to helping patients continue living independently after a stroke, caregivers can also help offer emotional support during this time. When someone suffers from a stroke, they are not only suffering from the physical effects of the injury but also experiencing changes in their brain structure and function. This means that they may have difficulty with basic functions like walking or talking, but it also means that they may have problems with memory, thought processing, and understanding language.

Because of this situation, having a caregiver who can help the patient adjust to these changes can be incredibly beneficial for them.

How to take care and advocate for someone with a stroke?

If you are caring for someone after a stroke, you can do a few things to make their recovery as seamless as possible. You should first keep their environment comfortable, clean, and safe, so they do not get confused or disoriented. Stroke victims have trouble moving around and getting around, so it is important to let them rest as much as possible. Patience is a virtue, especially in this case. It may be annoying to wait for an elderly person to cross the street or for them to maneuver around their house, but your impatience could be causing them unnecessary stress and frustration. For this reason alone, we should be more patient in these situations—and respect the elderly because we don't know what they have been through.

Some other ways to deal with patients with strokes include:

- Help them eat by serving up food that they can easily manage, like soup, fruits, or cereal.

- Ensure they have the proper medication prescribed by their doctor. Ask if they need any additional help with medications or treatment (such as physical therapy). If so, make sure they get it.

- Communicate openly, even if it means being honest about how hard things are sometimes.

- You must take it slowly and easily when caring for someone with a stroke. Moving around too quickly will cause more problems for them than good.

- If they are experiencing confusion, take care not to turn or move their heads abruptly.

- If they are having trouble speaking, it is best not to try to talk with them unless they ask for help.

- If they have trouble seeing clearly, it is best not to let them drive and monitor them until they recover their vision.

- Be aware of their level of consciousness. If they seem like they might be slipping into a coma, contact the medical team immediately so that you can make sure they receive proper medical care and get them to an emergency room if necessary.

- Encourage them to talk about what happened when they were injured. If possible, encourage them to write down their thoughts or feelings about what happened so that doctors will understand why they are experiencing difficulty.

- Keep a list of emergency contacts in your wallet or phone, so you can easily reach out if necessary. This list should include police, doctors, nurses, social workers, and other emergency services personnel.

How to take care of yourself while caring for someone with a stroke?

When caring for a patient with a stroke, it is important to be aware of how your mental health may be affected. You could be doing everything in your power to help them as much as possible. But sometimes, all the love in the world can't fix everything or help them get better as fast as they need. Here are some tips on how to take care of your mental health while caring for a patient with a stroke:

- Make sure you have enough time to get things done. If you are feeling overwhelmed, try delegating responsibilities or asking people for help.

- Be patient and compassionate with yourself. Sometimes it can feel like you are doing everything right, and your patient still has problems. Be kind to yourself when this happens, and remember that sometimes what we see as a failure is actually just the beginning of something great.

- Do things that make you happy. Studies have shown that even simple activities like knitting or reading can help improve moods when done regularly. So do not feel guilty about spending some time with yourself—you are worth it!

Focusing on the patient's needs can be difficult when you are worried about your own. You can do this by keeping a journal or diary of your thoughts and feelings about the situation. This will help you to process what is going on in your head and give you an outlet for all those emotions that are just bubbling under the surface. You could also try meditation or mindfulness exercises to help you stay calm and focused during this time. These practices can help reduce stress levels, which will help make it easier for you to manage any emotional issues that may arise while caring for someone with a stroke.

Finally, do not forget to take some time away from the situation so that you can clear your head and relax. Your selfless acts are what make the world a better place for people with the illness to feel content, and you should be grateful to be in that position where their lives depend on you.

Key Takeways:

- Strokes cause brain cells to stop working normally by depriving them of oxygen.

- Symptoms include loss of muscle control, paralysis, and difficulty speaking or understanding speech.

- The causes of stroke are high blood pressure, smoking, diabetes, and high cholesterol levels.

- A person with a stroke will go through five stages of recovery. Each stage has varying symptoms.

- A caregiver can help a person recover from a stroke and help them live independently.

- Advocating for patients with strokes includes patience, understanding, and providing both physical and emotional support.

CHAPTER 10

Caring For Caregivers

~~~

Caregivers are the backbone of the healthcare system. They play a vital role in providing support in the lives of the elderly, rain or sunshine; they are known to have the strongest personalities due to their work. Hence, tendering for caregivers is critical to ensuring that these individuals have access to information, resources, and emotional support when they need it most. It is also essential for helping them maintain their health and well-being while they care for the elderly with illnesses.

How can family members help a caregiver that is taking care of their loved one?

Supporting caregivers is vital because they make sacrifices to care for others and sometimes their own health. We must understand the impact this has on them and their families, so they can feel supported and cared for. Family members can help a caregiver by providing emotional support and physical assistance, as well as offering financial assistance.

Financial assistance is always essential in helping someone take care of their loved ones in any situation, especially for caregivers who may not have enough money. A caregiver's income will depend on how much time they spend with their patient and whether they have other responsibilities like work or school. Suppose there are other expenses associated with taking care of the elderly, such as transportation costs or medical bills. In that case, money might not be enough on its own to cover these expenses alone. Hence, providing financial assistance can help lessen the burden of the caregiver's expenses.

The best way for family members is to first ensure that the caregiver has all the information they need to care for their elderly loved one as they frequently check on their caregiver's mental health. This includes:

- Keeping the caregiver's basic needs a priority.

- Being there for them when they are feeling gloomy and supporting them during difficult times.

- Helping the caregivers figure out what they need and how they should be doing things.

- Ensure the caregiver has access to all the information they need, so they do not miss anything.

- Set time aside for your caregiver to talk about their experiences and feelings. This will help them feel heard and understood, which can make them more confident in their ability to care.

Family members should also be willing to do small tasks at times for the caregiver—like setting up a system for arranging groceries, providing household chores, such as cooking meals or cleaning up after meals, or managing medications—so that the caregiver gets a break from their difficult duties.

How can a caregiver use self-love to better care for themselves and avoid caregiving burnout?

Caregiver burnout is a state of physical, emotional, and mental exhaustion. You may feel hopeless, helpless, and isolated. You may also have trouble sleeping, concentrating, or not having the energy to do anything. If you're at risk of burning out, there are some things you can do to help yourself. The findings of a qualitative study conducted by Furlong on caregivers' mental health found that caregivers felt undeserving of self-care, and their demands for self-care were not viewed as vital by those for whom they provided care. Many caregivers lose motivation when they avoid self-care practices and building meaningful relationships. That is why it is essential to keep the caregiver's health in check to avoid burning out or developing depression on the journey.

The first thing caregivers should do is to keep their health a priority by incorporating self-love practices. Taking care of yourself is just as important as taking care of others, so make sure to occasionally put your needs first. According to psychology, self-love is the practice of taking care of yourself emotionally and mentally. It includes making decisions that nurture your mental, physical, and emotional health. It looks different for everyone, but some examples include setting boundaries, saying no when needed, taking time for yourself, investing in supportive and supportive relationships, doing things that make you feel good, eating healthy foods, and exercising.

Practicing self-love can be hard because we live in a society that often teaches us to put others first and not value ourselves. However, it is so important to do things that make you happy because if you don't, who will? When you practice self-love, you are filling up your cup so that you can pour into others from a place of overflow rather than depletion. Additionally, people who love and value themselves are more likely to be successful and have fulfilling relationships.

Most people think of self-love as selfishness. However, loving oneself doesn't mean that you are narcissistic or egotistical. It simply means that you regard yourself with kindness and respect. It is an essential part of a healthy lifestyle. Though it might seem selfish at first, self-love is essential for living a happy and healthy life. When we take the time to care for ourselves, we're better able to show up for others in our lives. We're also more likely to make choices that support our overall well-being instead of harmful or detrimental choices.

The more self-love practices you incorporate into your life, the happier and more positive you will feel. Self-love is integral to a healthy life, whether you're feeling stressed, sad, or anxious. In fact, research shows that self-love has many benefits:

- It helps you sleep better.

- It improves your mood and outlook on life.

- It reduces your risk of depression and anxiety.

- Symptoms of chronic illness are reduced.

If you are not sure what to do, here are some tips:

- Get yourself a support system. It could be family or friends, people who know what you are going through and who can help you if things get overwhelming.

- Know your rights as a caregiver. You may be able to receive health insurance benefits from Medicaid or Medicare. If you live in a state that offers long-term care programs, additional benefits may be available to help cover your expenses.

- Keep track of your expenses and ensure you stay within your budget. This will help ensure that you do not run into financial trouble because of caring for an elderly relative or loved one with special needs like dementia or Alzheimer's disease.

- Exercise is known to help with feelings of depression and loneliness while improving your mood and ability to cope with difficult situations.

Eating well-balanced meals will keep your blood sugar stable so that you don't feel tired or exhausted all the time.

Taking time for yourself does not mean spending all day answering calls or text messages from your loved ones who may be worried about your well-being but finding ways to recharge your batteries and relax after hours of caring for the elderly. Being able to spend time with people who are not part of your family makes it easier for caregivers to pursue their own interests, hobbies, or relationships outside the home.

Finally (and perhaps most importantly), caregivers should make time for fun. This may seem counterintuitive at first because we think caregiving is very stressful - but it does not have to be. You can still enjoy things like movies or games without feeling guilty about taking up so much time when they help keep you entertained.

What is self-care?

Self-care is the practice of taking care of yourself both physically and mentally. It can be something as simple as taking a bath or as complicated as a skincare routine. Self-care is caring for yourself in ways you would not otherwise have time to do. It is about taking time out of your day to look after yourself, so you can be your best at work and at home.

When you feel like you are not getting the support you need, it can be hard to stay motivated or even get out of bed in the morning. When you are feeling overwhelmed, self-care is something that can help keep things in perspective and give you the energy you need to continue. Self-care also helps you have a better relationship with yourself—you will be more at peace with yourself and keep those around you feeling happy.

It helps you feel better when you are struggling with depression, anxiety, stress, or other mental health issues. On top of that, it helps prevent mental illness from getting worse. Self-care allows you to be in a state of mental and physical equilibrium, which means that when you go to work or start a new project, you will be more focused and able to get things done. At the end of the day, when you come home from work, you'll feel more relaxed and ready for the next thing.

The best part about self-care is that it does not take much time at all—just 15 minutes if that—and it can be done anywhere and anytime. You do not need special equipment or fancy spa treatments; all you need is some "You Time." Self-care is not just the act of taking time out to relax, but it can also include doing things that you enjoy and find relaxing.

So, the question is, how do you know what you enjoy doing?

It could be small things like going for a walk or taking a hot shower before you get dressed in the morning, or bigger things like meeting up with an old friend, shopping or eating out at a fancy restaurant

Find out what works best for you because anything that puts you in a state of happiness can be your self-care moment. If it makes your heart flutter, it's probably worth it. Self-care is a way to control your life and ensure you are doing things that help you live the best life possible for yourself.

Tips for self-care

Self-care can seem like a luxury when you're juggling a million things at once, but it's essential to maintaining your health and well-being. Taking even a few minutes for yourself each day can make a huge difference in your well-being. Here are a few simple tips on how to incorporate self-care into your busy schedule:

- Talk about what is bothering you: Expressing your feelings is one of the best ways to relieve stress and tension in your body.

- Get enough sleep: Most adults need around 7–8 hours of sleep per night. If you're not getting enough rest, you'll be more prone to illness and stress. Make sure to prioritize sleep by going to bed and waking up at the same time each day and avoiding using electronic devices in bed.

- Go outside and enjoy nature: Get some fresh air and clear your mind by connecting with the nature around you. It doesn't matter if it's raining or snowing—just go outside.

- Find an activity that makes you feel strong and empowered. Maybe it's yoga or running around the neighborhood with friends? Whatever it is, find an activity that makes you feel stronger than ever before.

In the end, being a caregiver isn't always easy; it requires a lot of patience and mental toughness. Self-care is important, and you shouldn't feel guilty if you don't feel like meeting up with a friend one day or forget to go for a walk or to the gym. But with time and practice, you'll discover the unique value of this experience - and appreciate that it offers you the opportunity for self-discovery and personal growth.

Key takeaways

- Self-love is helping yourself to feel good—from taking time for yourself to doing things you enjoy to putting yourself first.

- Self-care is caring for yourself in ways you would not otherwise have time to do. It is about taking time out of your day to look after yourself, so you can be your best at work and home.

- Find out what works best for you in whatever keeps you in a state of happiness, which can be your self-care moment.

- Carving out even just a few minutes each day to focus on yourself can make a huge difference in how you feel.

Conclusion

Caring for and nurturing the elderly is important to communicate love, compassion, and respect. It is essential to understand that older people can be resistant to changes in their environment but respond well to care when they receive it. Caring for elderly parents is a mandatory obligation that all children must strive to fulfill. The process of caregiving includes maintaining dignity, promoting mental health, and supporting mobility. All of these actions contribute to the ability of older people and their families to live fulfilling lives.

We live in a time when the success or failure of one's life can depend on a person's health and overall well-being. Societies have begun to recognize the potential benefits they can derive from the care and well-being of their older citizens. Governmental and non-governmental organizations have begun to address these issues and find solutions to them. Certainly, we are still a long way from perfecting the technique, but we hope that the world will become a better place for all of us as more steps are taken toward providing the best possible care for our older citizens.

So, overall, caregivers need to ensure that the elderly have a positive outlook on life and a positive relationship with them. It should be a goal not only to show compassion and respect but also to accept that the elderly are no different from us. With their years of experience, some wisdom, and perhaps a history of hobbies or passions similar to ours, it is possible to relate to them as if they were old friends. Then, as the dialog grows, they can become useful resources for each other.

Therefore, it is necessary to have a support system such as relatives, friends, or professional caregivers to better manage the lives of the elderly. Caring for an elderly loved one is hard work, whether it is done at home or in a specialized care facility. But with the right training, resources, and support system, more and more families are finding that they can stay close to their loved ones while living a full life.

The caregiving profession is a noble role that requires exceptional qualities that are hard to find in average people. Caregivers have compassion, great empathy, and a great love for others. Most importantly, they are able to listen to people's needs and wants when it comes to their health care. They listen and can effectively translate it into actions that their loved ones or assisted living facilities should take. With the booming trend of assisted living, caregivers are needed more than ever. Older people would not be able to reach their full potential without caregivers. Caregivers accompany the golden days with love and purpose, making their profession an integral part of society.

About the Author

The author is a rising star in literary creativity and the art of writing, a true multi-talent in his field, and a multi-faceted personality. Abijah Manga is originally from Africa, specifically from the Democratic Republic of Congo. He deals with society's spiritual, social, and educational issues in his works. Abijah Manga's writings attract readers' attention mainly because of their individuality, spontaneity, openness, and youthful freshness in the perception of current and contemporary reality.

Abijah Manga is an outstanding entrepreneur, a successful coordinator of youth programs, a professional interpreter, an expert in foreign affairs, and a gifted teacher; the sphere of his interests and preferences are diverse and multidimensional. Abijah is the CEO of Loving Home Care LLC and MIB Consulting LLC and also the founder of the Mabij Foundation - a non-profit organization dedicated to ensuring that marginalized children and people with disabilities in Congo receive a quality education. Abijah's desire to address social challenges and fight the effects of poverty was the motivation for opening his business.

Abijah's mission, ideology, and philosophy are to *"release wealth, reveal the richness of the soul, realize the inner potential, and utilize available opportunities based on altruistic and humanistic aspects, regardless of the individual's (in)abilities."* Abijah actively supports the integration of modern values with traditional beliefs. He believes in teamwork to foster the development and engagement of young people. The path to success, recognition, and honor was paved for the author through a challenging, winding, and complex life journey. Personally faced with the consequences of poverty, Abijah found in himself a calling to contribute a part of himself and his work for the good of society, from simple tasks to leadership positions. In fact, the author's mission does not end with the above deeds but only continues in a more effective, productive, practical form.

Abijah writes this book intending to educate caregivers and family members on how to best care for the elderly who are struggling with illness - with ultimate compassion, respect, and love. Abijah observed how older people were not treated fairly in society and in the community. To combat these negative attitudes, he established a special home care agency to help empower the elderly and enable them to live comfortably by relieving them of personal worries and providing emotional support so they can live their lives to the best of their abilities.

Abijah MANGA

Abijah believes that everyone deserves to be treated with dignity - especially the elderly who need proper care. He quotes, *"My mission is to inspire people to live their golden years with passion and enthusiasm. We can make a difference by caring for each other in our homes, giving them the attention they deserve, and ensuring we create a space where they can flourish and be their true selves."*

Acknowledgment

This project would not have been possible without the help of current and former clients of Loving Home Care LLC. I have learned a lot from them. I would like to recognize the invaluable assistance of Loving Home Care's employees, PCAs, LNAs, LPNs, and RNs. I am very grateful to:

DAVID, DEBORAH, GIFT, MICHAEL, ALPHA, KOJO, BETH, GARY, MONETTE, DIONNE, SHANTELL, CORINNA, AMINATA, JACOB, ASHLEY, BONITA, DOMONIC, KELVIN, ANDREA, HALIMO, MAJA, SARAH, ALTHIA, CELINE, SARA, GODELIVE, LETITIA, FATOUMATOU, JOACHIM, ALFRED, ESPERANCE, SALMATHA, CYNDIA, COMLAN BLANDINE, SAMANTHA, SHANEALL, BAFFOUR, AMPONSAH, CORI, LINDA, AMANDA, LIZEBI MOTELU, SARAH, ALIOUNE, MEGNISSE, GODELIVE, LETITIA, RICHY, MANGA OPERE JOHN CAMILUS, FATOUMA, SALMATHA, CHRISTELLE, WENDY, STEPHANIE, JEFFREY, ELLA, ROZE, EDNA, KWADWO, JAILYN, JEFFREY, CHRISTELLE, ELLA, GRACE, JEROME, LANLENOU, LAXMI, ADDAE, SHANTEL, FAVOR, HALIMAH, DENNIS, VIDA, THONTIN, BRENDEEN, BEBETO, MWANZA,

Abijah MANGA

LARBI, BARBARA, PHIONA, BAILEY, SHENNELLE,
PATIENCE, KALYCIA, LOLA, BENDAH, ALYSSA,
ESTHER, ELIJAH, CHARLOTTE, SHELLY,
CALYSSIA, JASMINE, SANDHYA, SAMANTHA,
VANESSA, DIOP, MONIQUE, JEAN MICHEL,
EKUMU, DESMOND, JENNIFER, SHANIQUE,
HAWA, SANDRA, BRIAN, HELIA, HILL, HILO,
ESTHER, NURTO, JEANINE, ALAIN, MOSES …

References:

1. Centers for Disease Control and Prevention. Chronic Kidney Disease Surveillance System https://nccd.cdc.gov/CKD. Accessed 2/19/2021.

2. Kidney Disease: Improving Global Outcomes CKD Work Group. KDIGO 2012 clinical practice guideline for evaluating and managing chronic kidney disease. *Kidney Inter.* 2013;3(1)(suppl):1–150.

3. Burrows NR, Vassalotti JA, Saydah SH, et al. Identifying high-risk individuals for chronic kidney disease: results of the CHERISH Community Demonstration Project. Am J Nephrol. 2018;48(6):447–455.

4. Stratton IM, Adler AI, Neil HA, et al. Association of glycaemia with macrovascular and microvascular complications of type 2 diabetes (UKPDS 35): a prospective observational study. BMJ. 2000;321(7258): 405–412.

5. Hoerger TJ, Wittenborn JS, Segel JE, et al. A health policy model of CKD: 2. The cost-effectiveness of microalbuminuria screening. Am J Kidney Dis. 2010;55(3):463–473.

6. National Institutes of Health. Health Information: Chronic Kidney Disease website. https://www.niddk.nih.gov/health-information/kidney-disease/chronic-kidney-disease-ckdexternal icon. Accessed 2/19/2021.

7. Chen TK, Knicely DH, Grams ME. Chronic Kidney Disease Diagnosis and Management: A Review. JAMA. 2019 Oct 1;322(13):1294-1304. DOI: 10.1001/jama.2019.14745. PMID: 31573641; PMCID: PMC7015670.

8. Feigin VL, Brainin M, Norrving B, et al. World Stroke Organization (WSO): Global Stroke Fact Sheet 2022. International Journal of Stroke. 2022;17(1):18-29. doi:10.1177/17474930211065917

9. Feigin VL, Nguyen G, Cercy K, et al.; The GBD 2016lifetime risk of stroke collaborators. Global, regional, and country-specific lifetime risks of stroke, 1990 and 2016.New Engl J Med2018; 379: 2429–2437

10. Boehme AK, Esenwa C, Elkind MS. Stroke Risk Factors, Genetics, and Prevention. Circ Res. 2017 Feb 3;120(3):472-495. DOI: 10.1161/CIRCRESAHA.116.308398. PMID: 28154098; PMCID: PMC5321635.

11. Pearson TA, Palaniappan LP, Artinian NT, Carnethon MR, Criqui MR, Daniels SR, et al. American heart association guide for improving cardiovascular health at the community level, 2013 update: A scientific statement for public health practitioners, healthcare providers, and health policymakers. *Circulation.* 2013;127:1730–1753.

12. Furlong KE, Wuest J. 6pSelf-care behaviors of spouses caring for significant others with Alzheimer's disease: the emergence of self-care worthiness as a salient condition. *Qual Health Res.* 2008;18(12):1662–72.

13. Kim Y, Carver CS, Cannady RS. 6pCaregiving Motivation Predicts Long-Term Spirituality and Quality of Life of the Caregivers. *Ann Behav Med.* 2015;49(4):500–9.

14. Johnell O, Kanis JA. An estimate of the worldwide prevalence and disability associated with osteoporotic fractures. Osteoporos Int. 2006;17(12):1726–1733.

15. NIH Consensus Development Panel on Osteoporosis Prevention, Diagnosis, and Therapy. Osteoporosis prevention, diagnosis, and therapy. *JAMA.* 2001;285:785–95.

16. Salari, N., Ghasemi, H., Mohammadi, L. *et al.* The global prevalence of osteoporosis in the world: a comprehensive systematic review and meta-analysis. *J Orthop Surg Res* **16,** 609 (2021). https://doi.org/10.1186/s13018-021-02772-0

17. Sözen T, Özışık L, Başaran NÇ. An overview and management of osteoporosis. *Eur J Rheumatol.* 2017;4(1):46-56. doi:10.5152/eurjrheum.2016.048.

18. Wright N.C., et al. (Nov. 2014). The Recent Prevalence of Osteoporosis and Low Bone Mass in the United States Based on Bone Mineral Density at the Femoral Neck or Lumbar Spine. *Journal of Bone and Mineral Research, 29*(11), 2520-2526. DOI: 10.1002/jbmr.2269.

19. Wysowski, D.K. & Greene, P. (Dec. 2013). Trends in Osteoporosis Treatment with Oral and Intravenous Bisphosphonates in the United States, 2002-2012. *Bone, 57*(2), 423-428. DOI: 10.1016/j.bone.2013.09.008.

20. Hasselgren, C., Ekbrand, H., Halleröd, B. *et al.* Sex differences in dementia: on the potentially mediating effects of educational attainment and experiences of psychological distress. *BMC Psychiatry* **20,** 434 (2020). https://doi.org/10.1186/s12888-020-02820-9

21. Report: 2022 Alzheimer's Disease Facts and Figures in the USA

22. Vickrey BG, Mittman BS, Connor KI, Pearson ML, Della Penna RD, Ganiats TG, et al. The effect of a disease management intervention on quality and outcomes of dementia care: A randomized, controlled trial. Ann Intern Med 2006;145(10):713-26.

23. Voisin T, Vellas B. Diagnosis and treatment of patients with severe Alzheimer's disease. Drugs Aging 2009;26(2):135-44.

24. Grossberg GT, Christensen DD, Griffith PA, Kerwin DR, Hunt G, Hall EJ. The art of sharing the diagnosis and management of Alzheimer's disease with patients and caregivers: recommendations of an expert consensus panel. Prim Care Companion J Clin Psychiatry 2010;12(1):PCC.09cs00833

25. Harris-Kojetin L, Sengupta M, Lendon JP, Rome V, Valverde R, Caffrey C. Long-term care providers and services users in the United States, 2015–2016. National Center for Health Statistics. Vital Health Stat 2019;3(43).

26. Arrighi HM, Neumann PJ, Lieberburg IM, Townsend RJ. Lethality of Alzheimer's disease

and its impact on nursing home placement. Alzheimer Dis Assoc Disord 2010;24(1):90-5.

27. Colelo KJ. Who pays for long-term services and support? Congressional Research Service, In Focus, IF10343. August 5, 2021. Available at: https://crsreports.congress.gov/. Accessed November 22, 2021.

28. Harris-Kojetin L, Sengupta M, Lendon JP, Rome V, Valverde R, Caffrey C. Long-term care providers and services users in the United States, 2015–2016. National Center for Health Statistics. Vital Health Stat 2019;3(43).

29. U.S. Centers for Medicare & Medicaid Services. Nursing Home Data Compendium 2015 Edition.

30. U.S. Centers for Medicare & Medicaid Services. Your Medicare Coverage. Long-Term Care. Available at: https://www.medicare.gov/coverage/long-term-care.html. Accessed December 18, 2021.

31. Centers for Medicare and Medicaid Services. Original Medicare (Part A and B) Eligibility and Enrollment. https://www.cms.gov/Medicare/Eligibility-and-Enrollment/OrigMedicarePartABEligEnrol.

32. https://www.caregiver.org/resource/caregiver-statistics-demographics/

33. Zarzycki, M., & Morrison, V. (2021). Getting back or giving back: understanding caregiver motivations and willingness to provide informal care. *Health psychology and behavioral medicine*, *9*(1), 636–661. https://doi.org/10.1080/21642850.2021.1951737.

34. Greenwood, N., & Smith, R. (2019). Motivations for being informal carers of people living with dementia: A systematic review of qualitative literature. *BMC Geriatrics*, *19*(1). doi:10.1186/s12877-019-1185-0

35. Deci, E., Koestner, R., & Ryan, R. (2001). Extrinsic rewards and intrinsic motivation in education: Reconsidered once again. *Review of Educational Research*, *71*(1), 1–27

36. Abell, N. (2001). Assessing willingness to care for persons with AIDS: Validation of a new measure. *Research on Social Work Practice*, *11*(1), 118–130.

37. Natl. Alliance Caregiver. AARP Public Policy Inst. 2015. *Caregiving in the U.S.: 2015 report. Rep*, Natl. Alliance Caregiv./AARP Public Policy Inst., Washington, DC

38. Schulz, R., Beach, S. R., Czaja, S. J., Martire, L. M., & Monin, J. K. (2020). Family Caregiving for Older Adults. *Annual review of psychology, 71,* 635–659. https://doi.org/10.1146/annurev-psych-010419-050754

39. Unpaid eldercare in the United States — 2017–18 summary. An economic news release from the Bureau of Labor Statistics.

40. https://meetcaregivers.com/caregiver-certification-basics/

41. Schulz R., Vistainer P., Williamson G.M. Psychiatric and physical morbidity effects of caregiving. *J. Gerontol. B: Psychol. Sci. Soc. Sci.* 1990;45:P181–P191.

42. Czeisler M.É., et al. (2020). Mental health, substance use, and suicidal ideation during the COVID-19 pandemic — the United States, June 24–30, 2020. *Morbidity and Mortality Weekly Report.*

43. Bauer, R., Sterzinger, L., Koepke, F., & Spiessl, H. (2013). *Rewards of Caregiving and Coping Strategies of Caregivers of Patients With Mental Illness. Psychiatric Services, 64(2), 185–188.*

44. Bauer, R., Koepke, F., Sterzinger, L., & Spiessl, H. (2012). *Burden, Rewards, and Coping — The Ups and Downs of Caregivers of People With*

Mental Illness. The Journal of Nervous and Mental Disease, 200(11), 928–934.

45. Mayeux, R., & Stern, Y. (2012). Epidemiology of Alzheimer's disease. *Cold Spring Harbor perspectives in medicine, 2*(8), a006239. https://doi.org/10.1101/cshperspect.a006239.

46. Harris-Kojetin L, Sengupta M, Lendon JP, Rome V, Valverde R, Caffrey C. Long-term care providers and services users in the United States, 2015–2016. National Center for Health Statistics. Vital Health Stat 2019;3(43).

47. Grøntvedt GR, Schröder TN, Sando SB, White L, Bråthen G, Doeller CF. Alzheimer's disease. Curr Bio 2018;28:PR645-9.

48. Helzner EP, Scarmeas N, Cosentino S, Tang MX, Schupf N, Stern Y. Survival in Alzheimer disease: A multiethnic, population-based study of incident cases. Neurology 2008;71(19):1489-95.

49. WHO on China aging and health: https://www.who.int/china/health-topics/ageing

50. Goh, V. H. (2005). *Aging in Asia: A cultural, socio-economical and historical perspective. The Aging Male, 8(2), 90–96.* doi:10.1080/13685530500088472

51. Jaijagcomel W. Asia's aging population. In: The future of population in Asia. Honolulu, Hawaii, USA: East-West Centre; 2002. pp 83–95.

52. Goh VHH. Defusing Asia's aging time bomb. Health Affairs 2000;19(5):247–248. East-west Differences in Ageism

53. Vauclair, C. M., Hanke, K., Huang, L. L., & Abrams, D. (2017). Are Asian cultures really less ageist than Western ones? It depends on the questions asked. *International journal of psychology: Journal international de Psychologie, 52*(2), 136–144. https://doi.org/10.1002/ijop.12292

54. Ng, S. H. (1998). Social Psychology in an ageing world: Ageism and intergenerational relations. *Asian Journal of Social Psychology*, 1, 99–116.

55. Sung, K. (2001). Elder respect: Exploration of ideas and forms in East Asia. *Journal of Aging Studies*, 15, 13–26. doi:10.1016/S0890-4065(00)00014-1.

56. Palmore, E. (1975). What can the USA learn from Japan about aging? *The Gerontologist*, 15, 64–67. DOI: 10.1093/grant/15.1_Part_1.64.

57. Africa culture National Research Council (US) Committee on Population; Cohen B, Menken J, editors. Aging in Sub-Saharan Africa:

Recommendation for Furthering Research. Washington (DC): National Academies Press (US); 2006. 1, Aging in Sub-Saharan Africa: Recommendations for Furthering Research. Available from:
https://www.ncbi.nlm.nih.gov/books/NBK20296/

58. Abiodum, J.O. (2002). The Aged in African Society. Lagos: Nade Nigeria Ltd & F.B. Ventures

59. Lumun Abanyam, N. (2013, December 0). *The Changing Privileges and Challenges of Older People in Contemporary African Society - EA Journals.*

60. Abanyam, N.L. (2011). "The Problem of the Aged in Nigeria" Journal of Research and Contemporary Issues. Vol. 6 No. 1 & 2 America

61. Berger, R. (2017) Aging in America: Ageism and General Attitudes toward Growing Old and the Elderly. *Open Journal of Social Sciences*, **5**, 183-198.

62. Blakeborough, D. (2008) "Old People Are Useless": Representations of Aging on the Simpsons. Canadian Journal on Aging, 27, 57-67. https://doi.org/10.3138/cja.27.1.57 Europe

63. Rychtaříková J (2019) Perception of population ageing and age discrimination across EU

countries. Population and Economics 3(4): 1-29.
https://doi.org/10.3897/popecon.3.e49760

64. Walker A. (2005). A European perspective on the quality of life in old age. *European journal of ageing*, *2*(1), 2–12. https://doi.org/10.1007/s10433-005-0500-0 Aging

65. Jeste, D. V., Depp, C. A., & Vahia, I. V. (2010). Successful cognitive and emotional aging. *World psychiatry: official journal of the World Psychiatric Association (WPA)*, *9*(2), 78–84. https://doi.org/10.1002/j.2051-5545.2010.tb00277.x

66. Lin, Y. H., Chen, Y. C., Tseng, Y. C., Tsai, S. T., & Tseng, Y. H. (2020). Physical activity and successful aging among middle-aged and older adults: a systematic review and meta-analysis of cohort studies. *Aging*, *12*(9), 7704–7716. https://doi.org/10.18632/aging.103057

67. https://www.heart.org/en/healthy-living/fitness/fitness-basics/aha-recs-for-physical-activity-in-adults

68. https://news.utexas.edu/2019/02/20/interacting-with-more-people-is-shown-to-keep-older-adults-more-active/

69. DiRenzo, D., Crespo-Bosque, M., Gould, N., Finan, P., Nanavati, J., & Bingham, C. O., 3rd

(2018). Systematic Review and Meta-analysis: Mindfulness-Based Interventions for Rheumatoid Arthritis. *Current rheumatology reports*, *20*(12), 75. https://doi.org/10.1007/s11926-018-0787-4

www.ingramcontent.com/pod-product-compliance
Lightning Source LLC
Chambersburg PA
CBHW032055020426
42335CB00011B/349